M

how we live our
yoga

TEACHERS AND PRACTITIONERS

ON HOW YOGA ENRICHES,

SURPRISES, AND HEALS US

Personal Stories Edited by
Valerie Jeremijenko

Beacon Press, Boston

Beacon Press
25 Beacon Street
Boston, Massachusetts 02108-2892
www.beacon.org

Beacon Press books
are published under the auspices of
the Unitarian Universalist Association of Congregations.

Printed in the United States of America

05 04 03 02 01   7 6 5 4 3 2 1

This book is printed on acid-free paper that meets
the uncoated paper ANSI/NISO specifications
for permanence as revised in 1992.

Text design by Preston Thomas
Composition by Wilsted & Taylor Publishing Services

Library of Congress Cataloging-in-Publication Data
How we live our yoga : teachers and practitioners on how
yoga enriches, surprises, and heals us / edited by Valerie
Jeremijenko.
p. cm.
ISBN 0-8070-6295-2 (pbk. : alk. paper)
1. Yoga.   I. Jeremijenko, Valerie.
BL1238.52 .H69 2002
181'.45–dc21   2001001705

CONTENTS

introduction   1
Valerie Jeremijenko

coming apart in pune   8
Elizabeth Kadetsky

brick by brick   27
Samantha Dunn

the meaning of brahmacharya   36
Adrian M. S. Piper

lyric yoga   57
Stanley Plumly

the practice of paradox   67
Alison West

balancing acts: two views on ashtanga   77
Janet Bowdan and Roz Peters

an insomniac awakes   91
Lois Nesbitt

journey in yama-yama land   107
Robert Perkins

the art of breathing   120
Reetika Vazirani

how i became swami mommy   135
Judith Hanson Lasater

journey of a lifetime   142
Vyaas Houston

the guru question   159
Jeff Martens

subtle alchemy   173
Gladys Swan

corpse pose   181
A. B. Emrys

contributors   191

acknowledgments   195

introduction
Valerie Jeremijenko

Everyone who practices yoga has a story of yoga to tell. Whether that story is about the discovery of breath or the place of our long-time morning practice, whether it is about how yoga literally saved our life or about how it has subtly shaped it, we have stories of transformations and awakenings because yoga is that type of experience. It is an experience that moves us beyond our initial definition of who we are and puts us in touch with ourselves in a totally different way. It is an experience that stretches us beyond our limitations and invites our potential. While doing yoga we *eventually,*

are more ourselves, and more than ourselves. We sink into ourselves, and rise out of them. Yoga heals, nourishes, and challenges us. The practice infiltrates every corner of our lives. Some of us may develop on the yogic path enough to leave that sense of individuality and defining stories behind, but most of us won't, and for us the stories of how we live our yoga become a vital part of our personal narrative.

These stories have not been appreciated. In spite of the fact that literature—poetry, hymns, and epic narratives—has always been a traditional teaching tool of yoga, most of what is written today focuses on instruction, interpretation, or history. For those of us with a narrative cast of mind, who learn by connecting emotionally with others through their personal experiences, this means that many questions remain unanswered. Questions about how we can integrate yoga into our lives, philosophically, artistically, and logistically. Questions about what it means to make a commitment to the practice while living a contemporary Western life. Questions like, how is it for you? No; really, honestly, how is it for you?

This book is a collection of some of those stories and an attempt to address some of those questions. The authors—poets, writers, artists, and teachers—have different philosophies, levels of experience, racial identities, and professional interests. They all have different obsessions about their practice of yoga, and their essays naturally reflect this. Some focus on the role of teachers in their practice, others on the relationship of yoga to creative work. Some are critical of the institutional status quo of yoga, some share their miraculous stories of physical and emotional healing. And in their stories about their lives of yoga recognizable patterns emerge. These writers fall apart to come together, come together through falling apart. They step in and out of the moment, observing and reflecting. They embrace and confront. They open. Their essays analyze and investigate dissatisfactions and frustrations with the practice as well as understandings and experiences it has bestowed. The place of paradox, of restlessness and stillness, of acceptance and faith, all are examined in these pages with the unerring honesty and keen awareness that we like to associate with yoga.

I cannot overstate the importance of yoga in my life or of the evolutions and revolutions that have occurred in my practice. At first it was easy. For what now seems like a moment in the lifetime of my practice it was only yoga that defined my day. The rest fell into place around that central fact. If I had been asked at the time, I guess I would have said that the experience of yoga was about the experience of beauty: the beauty of the body in movement, of the early-morning quietness, of the breath coordinating with the rising sun. But my romance with yoga started in idyllic circumstances. I was traveling with nowhere to go. I was young and, I thought, free. On an island in Thailand I found Iyengar's *Light on Yoga* in the book box of a restaurant. Practicing on a platform in the sand I began to work my way through the week-by-week appendix. After morning practices I would read about the poses. After evening practices I would swim in waters bright with phosphorescence. It was a gift to start in such a place and to experience and accept such beauty. My body opened to it quickly.

And then I went to India, knowing nothing except that I wanted to know more. My experience of yoga in India was still about a romantic conception of beauty, and India offers many of those if that is what you seek. I remember practicing before dawn in Agra during Ramadan. The call to prayers, a woman preparing chapatis on a roof below, the sun rising on the Taj Mahal, and I surprising myself and luxuriating in the sensations of Urdhva Hunumanasana. Then Pushcar, the white city. Practicing on a hotel roof, still out of a book but for over an hour at a time by then. The trees that hung over that roof were home to hundreds of bats. Returning at dawn, they would carry water from the holy lake on their outstretched wings and splash it on me as I began my salutations. Finally, after months of practicing like this, I was directed to Mysore, where I began my practice again, this time in a semidark room of breath and gliding forms, of bodies flowing through contortions. They were incredibly beautiful, those forms and shapes. The light and shadows complemented them.

I was so confident of the place of yoga in my life after that. I remember saying "If you don't have time for yoga in your life there is something very wrong." But then I came to America and there were grad school, marriage, babies, our first jobs and un-employments. Then the joy of credit card debt and student loans, of a mortgage I still can't believe we qualified for. Ten years down the track my practice is very changed. If I think of beauty and romance in my practice now, it is only very briefly.

Which brings me to another question: Where are we as a nation in our romance with yoga? Is our heady infatuation over? Are we reaching a place where we can settle down to quietly dis-cuss it? I would argue that these essays suggest so. The writers do not seek or give instructions on asanas. Nor do they focus on tra-ditional philosophy to the exclusion of its context. They ask and attempt to answer what happens to a practice based on stillness and acceptance, in a world based on striving, distraction, and insatiable appetites. The cell phones in the practice room, our focus on achievement, the coffee we drink after class to get us up to speed again–all can modify how we view our practice and what we think we seek. All have the potential to pollute its very essence. Yet yoga is not supposed to be a monastic practice, or just a practice for the homeless ascetic. The yamas and niyamas are there to help us work out how we live our yoga while we live with others. Patanjali's Yoga Sutra II.33* tells us that the principles running contrary to our yoga must be investigated thoroughly. It tells us we must come to the practice through a study of opposi-tions and not through simple avoidance.

I read this sutra often. I read it and I try to practice it. I try to find the softness within the energy of my poses, the flight within my groundedness. I experiment with the point of imbalance within my balance, resist before surrendering. But the opposi-tion I keep on coming back to, the opposition I'd rather avoid, is the opposition of violence to nonviolence.

My daughters, ages six and two, sleep naked, intertwined in supta baddha konasana, their feet in prayer, their hips and knees falling open. When I watch them sleep I wonder if I could ever sleep like this. I wonder if I could put aside my knowledge of vio-lence, my fears and inhibitions, even with the most advanced of practices. I think not. And yet I know that nonviolence (ahimsa), in association with freedom from fear (abhaya) and anger (ak-

4

---

* I draw my interpretation of this sutra from Iyengar's *Light on the Yoga Sutras of Patanjali.*

rodha) are the very basic premises, the most fundamental practices without which my yoga is not yoga. But can I truly embrace them? Can I let the opposite go? When I watch my daughters sleep, which I do after a difficult time with bedtime or on days when I've lost my temper, I think back to myself sleeping as a child. I think back to the nights that I would climb into my parents' bed and fight against my siblings for a point of contact with my parents. For me the fight was harder than it has been for my children. There were ten of us, not two. On good nights, if I was lucky, I would be able to place my hands in prayer between my father's thighs and let the warmth soak through me. But I slept in a ball, as tightly curled as possible. It wasn't just because of space.

My parents were eccentric, foreign in small-town northern Australia, where any type of foreign was much too foreign, but good and loving people. My mother took in homeless people, my father laid the bricks and mortar of his church. But there were ten of us in fourteen short years and we were as wild as our parents' conflicting ideologies. My father was a refugee from Eastern Europe. In his church the men stood on one side singing, while the women, black lace on their heads, stood on the other and silenced the children. That was how my father wanted to live his life. But my mother was raised by maiden Irish aunts. Never switch on the toilet light. Never pick up a man's dirty socks. That's what the Aunties taught her. So in the midst of all the babies that were made and came and grew there were the bad nights, too. Nights when I would dig below the covers of my own bed, curling beyond tight, nights when I would run with a younger child in my arms and sleep in dirty laundry, nights when there was no hiding or sleeping. Of those I remember my father trying to choke my mother and the mass of children thrown to the floor while trying to protect her. Of those I remember being torn from our places one by one, and the welts on my brother's back. And yes, that was in another country and long ago, but still that violence is in my body. I feel it and I fear it. I feel it between my shoulder blades if I miss one day of practice. I feel it in my neck and head if I happen to miss two. And even with the

5

practice it doesn't always release. I can walk away from a two-hour practice with it still brewing on the edges. And I have turned it against myself in yoga too, so that now instead of the easy, fluid movements of the early days I have to watch my injuries carefully. It is my hips I hurt most recently.

And so I return to the sutras and read again, become nonviolent by studying violence. Invite the one by confronting the other. Avoidance is certainly easier and I would choose it if I could, but we choose only the battleground, not the battle we fight. We choose only on the basis of the sum of all our choices. The Bhagavad Gita teaches this. My parents didn't choose to live a violent life. They were good and loving people. But the way they positioned themselves made them vulnerable to going over with the overwhelm, over and over again. There were many things to push them. Too many children, too little time, too much work, too little help; too much stuff oozing from the closets, too much debt and the worries it brought them. But all those forces of violence are with us here and now. Our culture makes an art of inventing and propagating new forms of violence. Debt has a particularly American flavor as well, the result perhaps of so much craving—but that is to say nothing of the food we eat, the movies we watch, the structures and histories that define our lives, or of the pace at which we work and the guns many keep in their closets. Perhaps this is, in part, why Americans are embracing yoga so very fiercely now. Perhaps like me, they recognize that avoidance of violence isn't always possible.

I was bred to violence. There is a switch within me still. I do not know where it is or what exactly it will trigger, but it contains the energy to move me out of my body and beyond my self-awareness for long stretches at a time. And my anger can be so unreasonable, so undefined and nebulous. I acknowledge this and what it means as I watch my daughters sleep, so fearless and so innocent, with their sheets kicked off and their knees falling open to rest one upon the other's. I know that if they are to sleep like this, for a little while longer at least, that I will have to keep my awareness clear and always beware of the pressures I allow to crowd my life. And yet I also know that I am not the only one that harbors the potential for violence against them. It is there within us all, an untapped force in some, in control in others, fed into those with power from the moment they take breath. Knowing this, I wonder what I wouldn't do to stop my daughters from being among the one in four who might–no, will–be violated. And what does that mean to my practice? Is my practice of nonviolence sincere if I already foresee the circumstances under which I would reject it? Can I afford to use it as a weapon for protection? Do I really believe in the protection that it offers?

Perhaps the answers to these questions lie in the concept of nonattachment. Perhaps if I could nonattach, remove myself emotionally, I could accept the reality of violence without fearing its threat to my children. But I am not ready for this. In regard to my children I am Judeo-Christian and practice love, unconditionally.

And still I practice yoga. My practice leaves much to be desired these days. My morning practice was sacrificed long ago, first to nursing and then to the endless negotiations required to get my children out the door. Now I run away to practice at lunchtime, get illicit stretches in before, during, and after teaching, go through major family negotiations to get a Sunday practice in. I do this because the practice releases memories and tensions from my body, because it makes me feel like a safer, better person, and because as I sit beside my daughters sleeping I hope they will always sleep with their feet in prayer. This is how I live my yoga. The writers included in this book live it very, very differently. Many of them have entered realms I have been lucky enough to avoid. Many have already established that sense of distance that allows them to objectively observe. Some, like me, are at the beginning of the voyage and discovering the discomfort as well as the joys. All have taught me something surprising. I cannot begin to express my gratitude to them or my excitement at sharing their work with you.

Namaste.

coming apart in pune
Elizabeth Kadetsky

We practiced and took classes four hours a day, working in an airy top-floor studio where the sounds of Pune's hectic streets drifted in through the orange poinciana and neem trees, their leaves dangling over outdoor changing balconies. The school was a cloister far removed from the Indian miasma outside.

B. K. S. Iyengar was always present, twisted like braided bread into an advanced posture in the back of the studio. He situated himself between pillar and window, strapped himself onto yoga furniture, and meditated—often in the presence of a camera crew from Delhi at work on a documentary about the Iyengars–India's first family of yoga. From time to time, Iyengar quietly slid from his constraints and sidled up to a student to correct a flaw. The sound of his voice would attract the attention of all present who, upon gathering around him, inspired extended monologues and even demonstrations on the finer points of, say, how to straighten a leg.

His daughter, the yoga teacher and author Geeta Iyengar, could be found in the righthand corner of the studio, dressed in celibate's white and reposing in a restorative asana–she was not known for her active yoga practice. There she lectured to a coterie of international protégés, sometimes picking up a thread from the previous day's class. Her followers included a handful of Western women who had relocated to Pune several years back and took Geeta's word as the gospel on yoga for women. Sitting in similarly supine postures, they called across the space, discussing with Geeta the institute's latest publishing ventures, her upcoming travel schedule, and errors made in the blundering testimony of yoga students who had dared write up a workshop or lecture.

Iyengar's son, Prashant, a yoga teacher too, also had his devoted followers, and their practice time was also for meeting. They consisted mostly of Indian men, who gathered with him in the far left of the studio. There Prashant dutifully hung upside down for twenty or thirty minutes in either headstand or backbend, supported by a sturdy loop of rope that dangled from the ceiling. By his side stood his followers, conversing in a jumble of Marathi and Hindi about politics, Indian music, and Prashant's latest thinking on the Hindu classical texts.

Through this mix wove Pandu Rao, the institute secretary, barking into his cordless phone while walking it to either Iyengar or Geeta or Prashant, who dutifully responded to telephone queries from the equaniminous repose of yoga asana.

To me, one of those unaffiliated with any particular corner, the clearly defined social delineations sometimes seemed more like a chaotic overlapping of signs and signals–heightening my sense of the confusion and complicatedness on the Indian streets outside. I was spending as much of my two-month visit as possible walking and bicycling though town, attempting short phrases in the regional tongue, Marathi, speaking to store owners and rickshaw drivers, passing out cookies to the child beggars who clung to the pant legs of travelers chanting, "No mami, no papi, no rupee."

One day I was at the train station, where the misery and filth exceeded even that in the poorest slums in town. Children were tailing me–"No mami, no papi . . ."–and flies swarmed in front of my in the heat. Suddenly, a girl in a tattered sari ran to my front. She thrust a bandaged limb toward my face. It was leprous. A red globby substance oozed from the edges of the bandage and through gashes in the middle of it. One of those holes was dark, catching my eye. I stared, trying to make sense of it, when I saw movement inside of it. Flies obscured what I was seeing, but finally I understood. The gash was infested with maggots. The girl looked at me with a theatrical expression of misery, something masking whatever she truly experienced. I turned, and I fled.

Since I'd made the journey from the Bombay airport to Pune several weeks earlier, I'd become skilled in rushing through public places so as to keep a bearable distance from the misery all around. But suddenly my eyes became unshielded. I was losing the ability to assimilate the rigors of the street in India. It seemed I no longer possessed that practicality that allowed me to ignore the irreconcilable differences between those on the streets and those I knew at the school, between those on the streets and me. Now I could not make this world coherent. It was invading my dreams, waking me with nightmares.

In the intense environment of the yoga studio, and with the strenuous physical and mental work of developing asanas, I understood more than ever my need to make myself, unlike the world outside, cohere into a rational whole. Three years before, I had suffered from a kind of fragmentation of mind and body that culminated in a severe case of anorexia. Coming to India to study the mind-body therapeutic technique of B. K. S. Iyengar seemed a way to bring those parts of myself together again, to rejoin mind and body in the process of healing those emotional rents that had taken physical form inside me.

But now, I wondered if I was moving further from the goal. I was experiencing a kind of dissolution. In practice and in daily classes with my teacher, Geeta–who was not known for her "bedside" teaching manner–I could see that I was becoming emotionally unshielded. In an environment where everyone was undergoing his or her own profound psychic and physical changes, it was easy to be trusting. At a certain point, though, I wondered if I had left myself too exposed.

When I'd arrived at the school, I'd found the institute tableau amusing, replete with a cast of characters who fit the curiosity that was Iyengar yoga. I realized now that the spectacle was not funny at all. I was learning, as everyone did, that it was impossible to forever avoid breaching rules when your upbringing did not prepare you for a culture as ritual laden as India's.

Away from the school, students groused. A friend who'd gone home sent me an account from the newsletter of an Iyengar yoga association in Europe: "People may think of or go to Pune expecting an immaculate jewel–certainly it is a jewel in the yogic crown but it is not immaculate," he wrote. He went on to narrate a class with Geeta identical to one I had witnessed several times:

> One day she was teaching . . . the nadi sodhana pranayama (one of those ones where you twiddle your nose with your fingers). This manipulation requires short fingernails to enable you to get the tips of the fingers into the correct position on the nose. Geeta found that not everyone had the prescribed length of fingernail and then proceeded to rant on about how people come to pranayama classes with long fingernails. Well true enough but nobody knew that we were going to do this pranayama. . . . Now would it not have been more reasonable to suggest that those persons who had long fingernails . . . could do say ujayi pranayama . . . ? It would not take much imagination to suggest this sort of solution to the problem, rather than the inelegant approach of shouting at people. After all shouting at people does not make their fingernails shorter.

I was not alone in erring daily, but solidarity made it no less painful. One day in Geeta's class, I searched for a space of wall on which to place the soles of my feet. The pose was Setubandasana, named for a historic bridge in India. In its Iyengar rendition, you lie on the ground, then lift your buttocks and rest them on a wooden block, and then straighten your legs so your feet press against a wall. The room was crowded, and I found only the marble base of the statue of, as it happened, yoga's progenitor Patanjali. I placed my feet against the marble. It was cool. Something did not seem right, but I was tired and lightheaded from an hour and a half of contortions. Claudia, a regular fixture in Geeta's coterie of Western devotees, came rushing, breathless. "Elizabeth!" she said, speaking in a heavy French accent. "You know the feet are unholy! On Patanjali! You soil the founder of yoga!?"

My feet were destined for missteps. Another day I placed a plastic bag on the changing balcony before I entered the studio to practice. The bag contained several objects I planned to give away, among them a pair of sandals that I'd bought but never worn because they didn't fit.

Halfway through a headstand, I heard a whisper from the balcony. "Chappals?"

The word then circulated the studio as in a game of telephone, whispered.

"Chappals?"

"There are chappals?"

The whisper grew to a conglomeration of increasingly frantic sounds, until finally Sarah, another of Geeta's acolytes, shouted from the balcony, "Who has brought chappals into the studio? There are chappals on the balcony!"

"Chappals?" I heard the word uttered more, and then, finally, the translation that had escaped me. "Sandals."

My sandals, unworn, untouched by feet, had violated the tradition we all followed of leaving our shoes outside. I immediately whisked the contraband to the steps outside.

The other students were sympathetic, among them a petite woman from Amsterdam who rolled her eyes conspiratorially. Lucienne was a slip of a woman—her boy's body and pale skin gave her a virginal look, accentuated by her attire: Like Geeta, she wore all white. Lucienne looked like she was about twenty years younger than she really was, like a child. I had gotten to know her at a party at another student's flat. That night she'd talked at length about the tray of food she'd brought: raw vegetables, sterilized. She'd spent the day preparing them. Lucienne, I suspected, was anorexic. Watching her in practice, I was struck as though I had seen a ghost. Lucienne, frail and white, looked like someone I had been once. Knowing her reminded me that a part of me was nearly gone now. There was someone inside me I'd exorcised.

After I got to know her, Lucienne arranged for me to take the flat she'd been staying in, a pleasant Raj-era monk's cell with foot-thick walls and painted shutters that looked out on a mango tree. On her last day at the school I would move in.

In practice, Lucienne did not count herself among the women who lay around Geeta in supine poses discussing institute business. Like me, she favored the more active asanas; I often marveled at her ability to arch her back into upside-down circles from which she could then lift either leg or flip up to standing. Today Lucienne hung from a ceiling rope, Prashant-style. No one was paying attention, really, when she came down. I looked up when I heard howling. Lucienne was standing on the ground, grabbing the ropes with her arms as her body went slack and dangled. She kept shouting, big sounds belting from small lungs. Then she crumpled to the floor. Several yoga students rushed toward her to arrange her body to rest.

Afterwards, Lucienne was shaky. She gave me a wiggly smile and said she was glad she was leaving Pune. Her smile crumpled in the same way her body had, her paper-thin skin shrinking like a page when you throw it on fire.

Later, Claudia told me Geeta was angry at Lucienne. Lucienne had been practicing asanas too strenuous for her constitution. She'd brought this collapse upon herself.

I thought about Lucienne a lot after I moved to her apartment. She'd left small jars of health food products and a container of bleach with which to sterilize raw vegetables. I threw them all away, trying hard to erase her shadow. I also thought about what Claudia had said. It disturbed me. If Geeta had suspected a problem in Lucienne's practice, why hadn't she intervened earlier? Was Geeta secretly analyzing the actions of all her students, not with the intention of helping but to discuss them in gossip with her assistants? Was she silently watching me, too, making little ticks in a mental notebook when I dared perform what she thought insalubrious?

I decided to take up the issue with Claudia. I knew that Claudia and Geeta were close, and that Geeta, who was rarely approachable in private, accepted messages through her assistants. I asked for Geeta's advice. If she thought my practice unhealthful, could she suggest a better one? Was there something she could recommend for me? I had had irregular menstruation since suffering from anorexia, and no amount of yoga had yet set right my off-kilter hormones.

"You want a sequence?" Claudia mused, her finger on her chin, her eyes assessing my body from toe to cornea. Her knowing look made me wonder if the topic hadn't already come up.

My practice consisted mostly of backbends and upside-down poses. I had developed my habit after many years' work with my teacher, Manouso Manos, who from time to time gave me specific suggestions about which poses to perform, how long to hold them, and in what order to do them. In Pune, I'd added several poses to my repertoire, and come closer to achieving others, but essentially my practice followed my teachers' advice.

I did not hear back from Claudia, though I noticed Geeta watching me sometimes in practice; she grimaced when I did backbends, said things to her assistants that sounded like my name. Was I imagining it? She was certainly willing to discuss others. She ranted in the open about what had happened to Lucienne. "Why she was doing all the backbends!? I knew something, I didn't know what exactly. Why she didn't speak?"

Lucienne's breakdown preoccupied us all. I'd seen collective, seemingly psychosomatic epidemics seize yoga classes before. I wondered if another collective something, something viruslike and prone to suggestion, would infect others. Was what happened to Lucienne a hint of more to come? Might it happen to me?

In practice, the private lives of the family unfolded before the increasingly present camera crew. The documentary was the project of a longtime Iyengar protégé designed for broadcast on national TV, and, they hoped, to help win the school a larger domestic following. The crew clattered in and out of the studio almost daily now. When their lights clicked on, so did Iyengar. In practice another morning Pandu told us to come out of our poses. The students gathered behind the camera. Iyengar began setting up the stage for a demonstration, barking out orders to staff and students. "Why no one helps!? Eh? The bench over there, get that!" Several students leapt to retrieve the prop. "No, not that! The metal, the red, yes!"

Finally, Iyengar stood before the camera, electric. The crew became silent as he moved from one backbend to another. He did the pigeon and the king's pigeon, the wheel and the scorpion. Between poses he seemed physically winded, shaking out his mane and huffing, but in each asana he was the height of equipoise.

He stood facing forward now, and slowly moved a single arm and a single leg until he had embodied yoga's most performative pose, Natarajasana, named for Siva, the god of dance. There is a famous photo of Iyengar in the pose. It was taken more than thirty years earlier, at the great icon of Indian aesthetics, the Taj Mahal. In it he balances on a ledge on a single leg. The other leg reaches from behind as in a dancer's arabesque. He holds the foot of that leg with an arm stretched from above his head; the other arm points forward. The pose expresses a geometric harmony, heightened by its framing before the symmetrical monument. Today Iyengar balanced in that pose. His body rang out with the harmony of its shapes. We all watched, awed at the grace of a body so aged—he turned eighty in the winter. There was a palpable electricity flowing through passageways in his limbs.

Then that electric current jolted. And then it halted. What had I witnessed? No one else reacted, until Iyengar did. His body jerked again. He released the pose awkwardly and quickly walked off the stage. As he left the studio, we all stood, stunned.

In a few minutes Iyengar sprinted in again, but he seemed flustered and unfocused. He stood on the stage and called out a few instructions, and then descended into the pose Hanumanasana, or the splits, named for the flying monkey-god Hanuman. I'd seen Iyengar do the pose before and appear to be flying. Today he merely sank. Abruptly, he pulled his body from position and bolted.

We didn't see him afterward. That week, the cameras shut down. There were no interruptions in the classes, no theory discourses in practice. Nor was there an official explanation. The school got quiet. Geeta seemed less antagonized in class, but her mood was no less black. Every afternoon it was hot and sunny, and then as instantly as Iyengar had ghosted from our sight, monsoon downpours made deafening dart noises on the corrugated metal roof of the changing balcony. In class, when the first drops stung the roof, I imagined they were someone walking into the studio crinkling a plastic bag with new purchases. As the drops thickened, they sounded like more people with more bags. I kept looking over to see if any of those people was Iyengar, but it was only the air getting thick, and the sky dark, and the rains leaking on our clothes.

In time, someone close to the family confided that what had looked to me like a jolt of current in Iyengar's body was in fact a jolt of the heart. Iyengar had suffered a heart attack. It had been minor, but he had been ordered to stay in bed for a month. No practice, no teaching, no fraternizing with the students who seemed the lifeblood of the incorrigible teacher and performer. Iyengar had overdone it. Iyengar had been felled by something inside compelling him to act against his better interests. Was it his ego, or simply the joy of expressing what he loved most, or both–the thrill of being watched by others? Iyengar seemed very human to me in those days. Every morning I walked into the studio and scanned the empty space of floor between pillar and studio wall, and I felt a pang. I missed him as I would miss my own father, someone very dear, and very flawed.

By now I had switched half of my classes to mornings with Prashant, Iyengar's son. Prashant was warm and winning, but it was easy to see his physical being as a symbol of the decomposition all around. Prashant still had the wandering eye he was born with. It lolled to the far wall as he spoke. Coupled with an ironic glint in his good eye, a mischievous twist to his lips and a habit of rolling his tongue in his cheek, his entire bearing took on an almost absurd effect. To add to this, Prashant had been the heroic survivor of a tragic and freak accident in the mid-1980s that left him with a mangled right hand and arm. Despite years of yogic therapy he could now use neither to much effect, which made it impossible for him to demonstrate poses or give adjustments.

17

Prashant compensated with sheer mental outrageousness. He taught something unlike anything I had experienced in the hundreds of Iyengar yoga classes I'd attended. Prashant would put his pupils in a pose, and then stand in the front of the room spewing philosophy. He would quote from the Bhagavad Gita, occasionally reminding us to watch each breath as "a feather brushes against the interior lining of the body." I liked Prashant. His physical instruction lacked the intense attention to the singularity of every inch of the body that his father and sister stressed, but in his discourses he arrived, in a different way, at the Iyengar message of listening to the bodily intelligence.

One day he told us to take Trikonasana, triangle pose, a standing pose that was not unstrenuous when done over time. He stood on the platform, surveying us. "Watch what is the state of mind when you are in that reflective phase of Trikonasana," he began. We were not yet tired. It was possible to listen to each word. "It is inward. Study how the mind should be in trikonasana as much as you study the physical alignments. Glimpse the Great Mind behind the mind. In yoga we get *instacy*, not ecstasy. When you have ecstasy, you dance with the joy. It is external. In yoga we do not dance. We stay inside." I was finding it hard now, after several minutes in the pose, to keep track of his words. But by listening more deliberately, it was easier to ignore my body as it struggled to hold the position.

"Which is the softest, most fluid part of us?" he continued. He grinned, with a little shy smile. "The mind!" he boomed. I followed his reasoning, and then couldn't, and then could again. "It does not take any time for the mind to do something. It is there as soon as it thinks about it, whereas the body takes some time. Do the poses with the mind!"

Prashant continued his discourse as he led us through backbends. "Do not get the craze! Backbends bring the delirium potential! You will become insensible if you allow the arousal of craze, you lose the sense of judgment. You become passionate. For yoga you require an ideal dispassionate knowledge, unbiased." My mind, challenged to keep alert, remained focused. I began to feel lightheaded, but in an unscattered way. My thoughts did not wander as they tended to in daily life and even during yoga, but remained locked on each of Prashant's words. I heard each word as a singular ingot of meaning. The space between the words was empty; I heard a bright ringing sound in the moments of silence.

Prashant now instructed us to find a ceiling rope from which to dangle in headstand. I walked to a rope, my body seeming to glide there. My legs carried me, but the rest of my being, inside and out, mind and muscles, was still. I leaned into the rope and flipped upside down. When I came upside-down I felt a torquing in my upper back—one I'd experienced before in yoga. It was someplace deep inside my shoulder. I did not feel pain exactly, only sensation. I could see my whole self curled up in the spot where I felt the torquing. It was like an animate creature inside me, calmed and sleeping.

Prashant's words continued, like a lullaby. "Let the mind be still, hold it in its single space. Do not wander." He kept us there a long time, and then instructed us to come down from the ropes.

As I stood, blood rushed to my head. Little spots of black gathered at the edges of my vision. I was dizzy—nothing unusual. Then the black spots lowered from the upper limit of my vision field, and crept up from the base of it. Then the two lines of black at either boundary thickened, and then they converged in the center so all was black. Then I felt my body convulsing. Something screamed out from my throat. It was an invisible part of me, one I'd heard in my nightmares since I'd been here. My vision fragmented into splinters of dark and light. Then I was on the floor. I felt my body shivering and my torso and head shaking with my sobs. When I opened my eyes a crowd of yoga students had surrounded me, and they arranged me so I could rest. Just like Lucienne.

Afterward, for several days, I felt as if my body had undergone a kind of separation. I walked around slowly, as if it were necessary to give each piece of myself time to keep up with the other pieces. I had come to Pune to make myself whole, but in the process I was coming apart. I had moved into Lucienne's flat, and now her own fracture seemed to be repeating itself inside me. Iyengar, too, had broken down. Broken. We were all breaking.

I talked to Prashant. I asked him what had happened to me in his class. "You fainted," he said, seeming unconcerned.

"But why?" I asked, pressing for more.

"Perhaps you have debility. Physical debility, mental debility. What I recommend is, you eat some ghee." Ghee was a thick butter substance used in great amounts in Indian cooking that I was not fond of. Ghee could cure me? I looked at him ironically, an expression he returned in kind.

But I did feel weak. I was beginning to get migraines. A colony of India's fabled amoebas seemed to be squatting in my intestinal track. I ventured to the room on the institute's ground floor where Sarah had set up the computer that was the institute's erstwhile publishing engine. This was where Sarah more or less ran, as a volunteer, all of the institute's publishing business and much of its day-to-day affairs as well; it was also a congregating place for the several longtime students whom I joined in volunteering secretarial labor to compile archives out of the family's many writings and speeches. I asked if anyone could recommend a doctor. Claudia wrote out the name of a homeopath. Sarah told me she knew of an ayurvedic doctor. Someone wondered how I felt about Western, allopathic, medicine.

Pandu wandered in, his ever-present cordless phone attached

like an appendage at his wrist. He looked at me with his doe eyes. "What kind of path you need?" he asked. "I find for you. But I know what you need. You want allopathy? Homeopathy? Naturopathy? No. I know. What you need is sympathy. I give you sympathy."

We all burst out laughing at Pandu's quip, but I wondered if Pandu didn't have it right.

Iyengar was still absent when it came time for me to leave Pune. I'd studied at the institute every day for two months. Iyengar had spoken to me and charmed me, and Geeta had, in her own indirect manner, taught me. It had not been a fruitless summer, but I wondered, Was this all there was? Geeta had never offered a sequence of asanas, and the integrity of my very being, despite the strides I'd made in my physical, intellectual, and emotional approach to the poses, now seemed more compromised than ever. The man I had come to learn from had pushed himself to breakdown. I had thrust myself into an institution whose very structures and students seemed on the brink of breakdown themselves. And then I, too, pushed my physical and emotional limits to the point where I, like so much around me, was coming apart. Was this what I had come for?

I saw Claudia in practice my last day. The studio was barren—with Iyengar's absence, many regular students had stopped coming; Geeta was busy caring for her father. "You're leaving then?" Claudia said in her French accent.

"Yes," I said.

"You know Geeta, she never gave you a sequence."

"I know."

"It's because she doesn't want to. She didn't say, but this is what I think."

"Okay?"

"You know it's because your practice, you are doing everything wrong."

Her words stung. I'd studied with dozens of accomplished protégés of Iyengar who had guided me specifically for years. Iyengar himself regarded me as worthy. I knew she was wrong.

"It's as if you've never learned Iyengar yoga," she continued. "What I recommend is, you start at the beginning."

I had practiced for thirteen years now. She sounded ridiculous.

"You take *Light on Yoga*, you know Guruji has sequences at the back for people who are trying to learn on their own. You start there. Start with lesson one."

This was my good-bye. Secondhand, whether through Geeta I couldn't know. I left the institute angry. I was uninterested in studying ever again with Geeta. And yet I still felt a strange elusive draw from this genius named Iyengar. I hadn't had a chance to say good-bye–I didn't want to end here.

I might have, though, had it not been for events on my return journey to the airport in Bombay. International flights tend to depart Bombay in the wee hours of morning, making the Udiyan Express or daytime commuter trains from Pune to Bombay inconvenient, dropping you at Victoria Terminus in the early evening at the latest and requiring a long, expensive taxi ride out to the airport. A far cheaper and more convenient route to the airport was via shuttle on the Pune–Bombay Road, a byway whose place in Indian lore was comparable to that of Highway 17 in Silicon Valley–the most overused but undermaintained "highway" in the nation. It was said to be a winding, two-lane old cow trail paved with speed bumps every hundred meters. Owing to a lack of urban planning and a population explosion in Bombay that had made a suburb out of faraway Pune, this small trail had evolved into a major commuter artery.

It was late August; the monsoon was still bringing rain in dramatic outbursts, but with larger intervals between each torrent. By the morning of my departure it had not rained for several days, meaning that the road between Pune and Bombay would be safe–except in the case of an unexpected, last-minute downpour.

Of course by afternoon it was pouring. It was too late to get on a train. My shuttle picked me up, inauspiciously enough, an hour late. We wended in the dark through slumlike, dirt-pathed villages on the outskirts of Pune picking up passengers. This took two hours. I prepared myself for the possibility of missing my

5 A.M. flight. As passengers stumbled from their hutlike structures, addled by covered-wagons-worthy loads of luggage, I watched dust turn to mud and slither into gullies that were quickly forming beside our wheels. One passenger, a woman wearing a Punjabi dress and with a bright, engaging stare, started the immediate drill that is par for the course upon meeting a foreigner. "And you are?" she demanded.

I was not interested. "American," I mumbled, looking back at my magazine.

The next passenger was a portly man wearing an ill-fitting suit; he carried a briefcase with the stitching coming apart. "Which country?" he demanded.

"America," I repeated, looking down to discourage further intrusion.

I was thinking about how I was bored of yoga, sick of Geeta, fed up with people saying "yes yes" when they meant "no no" or weren't listening to begin with. I was fed up with shoddy tailoring and sloppy housekeeping and stinking toilets and hundred-year-old roaches and talking to people with whom I could not communicate because of a lack of a common language—be they Italian or Russian yoga students or my Marathi-speaking neighbors. I was sick of the way locals said "ayy" at the end of their phrases in a way that meant "Sure, even though I have no idea what you're talking about," and I felt the pain in my sacrum and the first dizzying hints of a migraine. I was sick of India, of dirt in the air; amoebas in the water; chappals that caused blisters and blisters that drew foot fungus that prevented them from ever healing; hard mattresses and mosquitoes and rickshaw horns and pigs on the street and filthy sacred bulls with crooked painted horns and limbless beggars and lepers with damp bandages thrust in your face and mean little boys swatting at you for spare rupees and the fake smiles of merchants who longed for you to give them your dollars. I was sick of the isolation of my foreign language, the impenetrable wall of noncomprehension, the lonely symbol I embodied as a foreigner in India. I was aching to leave India, and thinking about how if this shuttle never traversed this makeshift pass, I might never get to.

Outside Pune, the highway stretching ahead was indeed little more than street, pockmarked by potholes, broken up by sharp, ninety-degree turns, made barely navigable by speeding Maruti sports cars careering from the other direction carting neatly dressed businessmen who stared at the pavement with Nintendo eyes.

This vista lasted only a short while, however, for it was only minutes beyond the slums of Pune before we had a flat. The driver cursed and swung open his door; a torrent of rain and mosquitoes flooded in. The buoyant woman in the Punjabi dress asked me what time my flight was. She settled back comfortably into her double bench and said that hers wasn't until 10 A.M. She began to crochet. The man with the briefcase nodded cheerfully. His flight was at noon.

I watched out my window as the driver kicked at the tire a few times before prying it loose. He walked to the side of the road and stuck out his hand, hitching. Soon he got on the back of a scooter, holding the tire so it made a large O on the seat behind him. I watched the O slowly disappear into the mist of rain and dark on the long road reaching out to Bombay. The O was like the shape of someone's mouth saying, "O, look at the mess you're in."

The road was now deserted. Without the driver's flashlight, the Pune–Bombay road was as dark as it was quiet. "Is he coming back?" I asked my shuttlemates.

The woman in the Punjabi shrugged, crocheting.

"Oh sure," said the man with the briefcase. "No problem. Just ten minutes." Soon everyone else in the bus was nodding at me, echoing with false smiles, "Just ten minutes madam. No worry. No problem."

Two hours later the driver had not returned. It was now eleven, and the trip to the airport was supposedly four hours in good conditions.

When the driver did return, tire perched behind him on the back of another scooter, I had given up all chance of making my flight. "Come down," he said to me. "Your flight is at what time?" I told him. "Come." Outside, the driver directed me and another man from the shuttle into a jeep, packed with young Indian men. "Who are they?" I asked.

"Please madam," the driver said.

"Where are they going?"

"Yes yes. Safe journey!"

A chorus erupted from inside the shuttle bus. My former fellow passengers all urged me inside the jeep; they sounded like paid promoters assuring me of the efficiency and good will of India. "Yes madam. Inside!" "Yes madam. Ten minutes only." "Your plane, you will get!"

I got in. I was the only woman. I was wedged in the middle of the back seat between two young men, one of whom shoved his thigh so close to mine it was nearly in my lap. The other leaned over me with a seedy grin. "Excuse me madam. Which country?"

"America," I offered, staring fixedly at the dark road.

We were silent for a long time, but the second man, a boy, really, was still watching me eagerly. "Because, madam, I am going to Chicago." He pronounced the *ch* as in *chuckle*.

"Good," I said.

Hindi film music blared loudly from the front seat. The Chicago-bound kid beside me began singing along, bobbing his head from side to side with the music. I slid my carry-on bag from my lap onto the seat between me and the boy on my other side, shoving his thigh away from mine. He snorted.

We passed through a town. A ragged sadhu clung close to the walls as he limped down the street. There were a woman, barefoot, and a dog, limping, blocking our path. The driver bleated his horn at them. I remembered how India looked my first day at the Bombay airport, and on the odyssey of train and rickshaw rides that finally led to my being deposited at the sanctuary of the yoga school, and I realized how I'd been shielded from that India ever since, ensconced in the protective confines of the yoga school, and how the world inside the yoga institute was very far from this world that was India.

Chicago Boy leaned over me. "Are you hungry?" he asked, his head still bobbing such that he seemed to be looking at me upside down. "We could stop for dinner."

"No time!" I cried, but then caught myself. I still wasn't sure who they were, but I suspected from other conversation in the car that the boy had rented this jeep to get him to the airport. The other men were his drinking buddies and a hired driver. The other shuttle rider and I had no more rights than hitchhikers. "If you're hungry I have food," I offered, my hospitable instinct surfacing out of desperation. I slid a tofu sandwich from my carry-on. Chicago Boy frowned at it.

"Ten minutes only," he assured me.

Shortly, we pulled into an outdoor garden restaurant in a hill town called Lonavla. I knew about Lonavla because it was here that one of the first Indians to popularize yoga asana in the twentieth century had built his "yoga hospital," Kaivalyadam–"land of freedom." Here, seminal science experiments proving the health benefits of yogic meditation were conducted. Chicago Boy had never heard of Kaivalyadam's Swami Kúvalyananda. He knew Lonavla as a posh retreat for stylish Bombayites. At one A.M. it was bustling with well-dressed and giggly yuppies. "You take food?" the other boy leered.

"No," I insisted.

"We buy you pop," Chicago Boy pressed.

I followed them inside. The other men from the car scattered at other tables, and quickly all were shoveling down large portions of chicken biriani and rotis. No one at my table talked until the food was done. Then Chicago Boy, wiping biriani grease from his mouth with the back of his palm, looked at me balefully. "Do you know Chicago?" he asked. Suddenly his eyes looked very big, and his face and body very small. He had light-brown eyes with dark ridges at the edges of his corneas and deep black shadow lines around his eyelids. His skin was very dark. He told me he was going to Chicago to take a job as a computer engineer. He'd lived in London for a year doing the same thing, and he didn't like London. One time he'd been walking down a street there and was surrounded by a group of fourteen-year-old white boys. They started throwing pieces of garbage at him and calling him names—"beast" was mostly what he heard—until he ran away.

"Tell me something," he asked, leaning forward to hold my gaze. "In U.S., how are the people? Are they friendly?"

At that instant I saw him in America, a young man with dark

25

skin and a foreign accent and every right to be welcomed. I felt, strangely, a surge of national defensiveness not unlike what my shuttlemates must have felt when I hesitated outside the jeep by the side of the Pune–Bombay Road. I didn't want Americans to make a bad impression; I didn't want him to meet one Chicago racist, and if he did, I wanted him to know there were people he could call.

"Some of us, yes." I gulped. He still held my gaze. I saw nothing challenging, nothing mistrustful, only the open face of a person starting out on a scary adventure.

Chicago Boy got me to my plane on time. When we got out of the van my shuttlemate and I offered to give him money to help cover the cost of the car, but he refused. "I was just trying to help out." He shrugged. I gave him my number and e-mail in the States and told him to get in touch if he had any problems. He was my goofy angel.

Something changed in me on that traverse to Bombay, through that tunnel that was the Pune–Bombay Road. I had come to India to do yoga, but in the process I had discovered a place where raw emotion and my volatile impressions made me feel alive. I was being drawn to India, to its contradictions and what seemed irreconcilable; to the way it defied coherence yet remained a functioning "whole" nonetheless; to the way that what repelled me one minute drew me the next; to the way I could swing volubly from feeling alienated to feeling welcomed with the warmth of family, welcomed by Mother India. I knew that to understand yoga, I needed to engage the country it came from.

And I realized that Iyengar called, not Iyengar the head of the yoga school or even Iyengar the yogi, not Iyengar the healer or Iyengar the magician or Iyengar, as he was known in Pune, the man of rubber. But Iyengar the Indian, Iyengar the patriarch, Iyengar the man who had made me feel welcome despite the sometimes distressing goings-on at the institute he'd built. Iyengar the friend, whose presence in my life I cherished, Iyengar who had welcomed me to his family.

brick by brick
Samantha Dunn

I used to make fun of yoga. I was an editor at a national fitness magazine and a blood-and-guts kind of exerciser; I didn't consider anything to be a serious workout unless I came away with at least one bruise or a strained muscle. I once even wrote in an article that only granola-crunching, Volkswagen-van-driving, Birkenstock-wearing noodle-necks–I did use the term *noodle-neck*–bothered with yoga, clearly because they couldn't hack a real workout. Of course, I had never actually practiced yoga;

"down dog" was just a command I gave my pug. That I lived to become a woman who knows her Iyengar from her Ashtanga and her Kundalini is something I am grateful for each morning when I put my hands together and begin my meditations.

Two years ago, I took my horse for a ride in one of the southern California canyons near my stable. I have ridden since I was old enough to sit in a saddle; this ride seemed no different than a hundred others, although on this day I was particularly stressed and preoccupied with the many things in my life that appeared to be going nowhere. When Harley balked at crossing a small creek, I was irritated and impatient. Being stalled on him was a sort of metaphor for everything else in my life.

"Don't be a sissy," I told him, jumping off to lead him through the water. "I don't have time to talk you into this."

Harley seemed content to have me lead him, but when I skipped over a stone to avoid getting my boot wet, he suddenly reared back on his haunches.

Even as I write this I recall the shock and surprise when the bony force of his knee hits my back, and the sickening feeling as I realize my 2,000-pound thoroughbred is jumping the water. And he's landing on top of me.

As his body pulled away I saw the flash of a steel-shod hoof as it struck downward. Then I heard the crack of something, loud as gunfire, and looked to see my left leg snapped apart like dry kindling.

Harley's hind hoof had just come through my left shin, cutting through the bones, muscles, ligaments arteries, and veins like a dull shovel. Three fingers' width of calf muscle and sinew formed a gristly hinge. I remember feeling above myself, observing the leg separate and unmoving at the side of a woman's body, which I recognized as my own.

I don't know how long I lay there before I screamed for help. Time had no measure. I remember thinking about a conversation with a friend of mine; it was like a home movie playing in my head. I was lamenting a string of bad luck that had seemed to come my way; she wasn't sympathetic. "God touches us with a feather to get our attention," she said to me. "Then if we don't listen, he starts throwing bricks."

My blood pooled around me. Harley put his nose to my face. I thought, the brick. Finally, this is the brick.

I was saved by a man named Edward Albert Jr., an actor whose handsome face and sonorous voice I recognized, a disorienting fact that made me think perhaps I was in fact already dead and had been sent to a special afterlife for Los Angelenos. He kept me from bleeding to death by pinching the artery with his fingers; his daughter directed the paramedics to us when they couldn't find the trail. Edward never let go of my hand as we waited for the medevac helicopter to take me to UCLA's trauma center. "Your life will change because of this," he told me, "in ways you can't imagine now."

The doctors told me basically the same thing, but they said it in a way that was meant to prepare me for life as an amputee. I had a grade-three, class-B compound fracture of the tibia and fibula. Only a class-C injury, a crushed limb, is technically worse, but the severity of my injury increased exponentially just because it was done by a hoof. There is one reason for that: the high risk of infection, further complicated by the fact that I lay in dirt and mud for more than an hour before the helicopter could reach me. A titanium rod was crammed down the center of my tibia to join the disconnected parts; it runs through my knee and ends at my ankle, bolted in place.

The doctors sounded definite in their report, and I had no cause to doubt them: they are excellent and well-respected orthopedists: Even if the bone united—and the chances were not good—the soft tissue damage was extensive. Infection could take the leg, and maybe even kill me in the process. A latent infection could occur even years down the line and, again, take the leg. Blood supply had been seriously compromised; I was told not to expect feeling in a large part of my leg; too many nerves and veins had been cut. I would walk with a limp and never run again, that was for sure; in fact, there was a very good chance my limb would be a stiff, unfunctional appendage even if no other complications arose.

The only bright news they brought was about the "wonderful" advances in prosthetics. I could run with a prosthesis, dance too, maybe. New prosthetics weren't bad looking, they said.

"You can even ride a horse with it," my regular orthopedist told me, his tone cheery. "In fact, you can run with a prosthetic, and you'll never be able to do that with your leg even if it heals."

"Wow, how appealing!" I answered sarcastically. The look he returned said clearly that I would have to lower my expectations.

It was under these prospects that I returned home to face months of lying in bed, waiting, it seemed, for my leg to fall off. I remember the silence in the house, and the click of the hour hand as it moved over the face of the clock. I had the feeling that I was shackled to something; the reattached leg was not me but an attachment to me, something other than, in addition to.

Finances required that I start working again, which was possible because I was lucky enough to be able to do all my freelance writing from bed. I received an assignment from a celebrity magazine to report on martial arts and yoga as "fitness trends of the stars," all of which I did by interviews over the phone. And then I contacted a certain Sikh yogi named Gurmukh Kaur Khalsa.

"Why don't you come down here?" was the first thing out of her mouth.

"I just have a few quick questions . . ."

"Oh, I hate to talk over the phone. It's so much better if I can show you," she replied.

I don't know why I didn't tell her that I had not been farther than the grocery store in six months, or that I walked with the aid of a leg brace and crutches, or that pain was constant despite the Vicodin I took every six hours, or that I felt exhausted regardless of the fact I slept fourteen hours a day. Maybe I was just too tired to argue. I got dressed; my clothes hung on me like laundry on a line. I drove the forty minutes to her house, as directed.

Even before she opened the door the scent of nag champa

wafted through the open windows into the courtyard. A statue of Ganesha stood near the entrance; I grinned at what I thought was a kooky little elephant. I couldn't remember the last time I had smiled other than to put on a happy face for visiting friends. When Gurmukh opened the door she didn't even bother with hello.

"What happened to you? Here, come, let's sit on my bed. You can put your feet up and have some tea," she instructed, and I followed this barefoot figure dressed in white down a hall.

I don't recall exactly what was said in the hour or so we sat on her bed. I do remember the way she expressed no pity for me, and I was grateful, because the pity I felt from others made me feel hopeless, as if my very essence as a person had been reduced. It was if she expected me to get well; it was just a matter of me choosing to do it. She told me she wanted me to take her yoga class the following day. I looked at her like she was crazy.

"People in wheelchairs can do Kundalini yoga," she assured me. "Even if you only do three minutes, those three minutes will help you. We always say, Begin where you are."

When I returned to the car, I sat gripping the steering wheel and cried. I felt like a wanderer who had just found shelter and, now safe, could admit how terrified I had been of the storm.

For my first Kundalini yoga class I positioned myself at the back of the room, crutches against the wall. Someone helped me sit on the floor, my bad leg stretched out in front. To begin we put our hands together in prayer pose, thumbs pressed to the center of the chest, and closed our eyes. I listened to the others as Gurmukh led them in the chant "Ong namo guru dev namo," which she said meant we were bowing to the great infinite wisdom found inside ourselves. It struck me that I had not prayed with my hands together since I was a child. I have never had faith in anything; a certain ironic stance is the religion of my generation X. But at that moment of pressing palm to palm, lowering my shoulders and inflating my lungs with a full breath, I understood what it is to pray with the entirety of one's being. It just felt good.

While I couldn't manage most of the class, I could do some of it, especially the breathing exercises and mudras that had us hold our arms in certain positions. We inhaled the word *sat*, and exhaled the word *nam*, which together mean "truth is my identity." In that class I experienced a sensation that is not unlike falling in love.

The brick that had fallen on me had led to this truth: My entire approach to my body and to fitness in general had been based on the concept of deficit. I thought of aerobics classes and how I had panted my way through movements just to give myself smaller thighs, pumping iron to shape my narrow back, dieting to lower my fat level. I had always approached my body as if it were a problem needing to be solved. Not only that, as a writer and journalist I had taken this posture into every health and fitness article I'd ever written: *There's something wrong with you, but here's how to fix it.* This attitude was not really different from the notion of original sin, forever reaching for an ideal we are constitutionally incapable of attaining. But here I was, truly broken now, weak, emaciated, yet in front of me this teacher was saying that just by the virtue of my being, I was complete. I always had been. The only thing I needed to do was honor that. It was the only thing I'd ever needed to do.

From then on, I was in her yoga class at least three days a week, sometimes four. I would have lived there if I could. I lived in a way I never had: I massaged my body with almond oil and took cold showers each morning before meditating for half an hour, I ate a largely organic, vegetarian diet to provide myself with as many nutrients as possible for healing, I saw a Sikh chiropractor and an acupuncturist, and I took supplements to support my immune system. Most of all I did yoga every day, even if it was just a simple spinal flex. In class, when others were in asanas I could not do, Gurmukh told me to hold the posture in my mind, mentally going through it.

"If your yoga teacher told you to eat peanut butter and stand on your head, would you do it?" my ex-husband joked, echoing the sentiment of other friends and family who weren't quite sure how to take my lifestyle shift.

The answer was yes. Of course I would take any of her advice, for one simple reason: I was feeling better. I was able to bend my knee—which had been traumatized by the surgery to insert the titanium rod—and actually sit in easy pose. I needed my crutches less and less, so much better was my balance. And in my regular medical checkups, my doctor was noticing a change: My wound was looking healthy, no signs of infection, and there was substantially less swelling in the leg than anticipated. I had movement in my toes, and was even beginning to rotate and flex the foot.

But what I was feeling on the inside was perhaps even more profound, although here I run up against the limits of my ability to express myself. To say that I felt more calm and more optimistic is one way to put it, but it was more than that. It was almost as if something inside me had been frozen and I was feeling a chipping away, a melting, piece by piece.

However, there was still the problem of bone growth in the break. In the next year I went through two more surgeries, one to take the screws out near my knee which then allowed the bone to shift down toward the break, and another surgery to replace the titanium rod with a larger rod in the hope that would stimulate growth. My doctor warned that the first rod was also nearing "failure rate," and if it broke my healing would again be in jeopardy.

But even after the surgeries, there was little evidence of growth, despite the fact that I was doing all I thought I could for my healing. A bone graft surgery was scheduled; they would take marrow from my hip and put it on the break. Even my usually stoic surgeon said it was a painful process; now my hip would need to heal, too.

The prospect was depressing. I continued with my yoga, which lead me to the healing meditation practice of Sat Nam Rasayan, which, very roughly explained, is where a practitioner meditates with you on your problem. During one session Hargo Pal Kaur Khalsa, one of America's few expert practitioners, told me to "release an intention into the universe." As I lay in corpse pose what looped through my mind was the image of Michelangelo's Creation painting, where God and Adam stretch to touch fingertip to fingertip.

Some weeks later Hargo Pal and Gurmukh took me to see Guru Dev Singh Khalsa, renowned in the Sikh community for his mastery of Sat Nam Rasayan. I don't remember much of the day, since I was stretched out in a kind of twilight that is not quite sleep and not quite meditation. If a room can be dense with mental energy, this one was, with fifty people sitting or lying, quiet as stones.

At a break I was introduced to Guru Dev, whom I expected to ask me about my leg. He didn't. He just wanted to know about my horse. I told him Harley had been a racehorse bound for slaughter when he was rescued by a woman, who gave him to me. I made a flip comment about me saving him, because broken-down racehorses don't have much value.

Guru Dev stopped me. "No," he said, "you did not save him. He saved you. He is your guru. You know what is *guru*? *Guru* means that which brings you from darkness into the light."

My pre-op appointment came, a few days before the bone graft surgery. It was just a routine check; I'd had X-rays less than a month before, so I wasn't scheduled to have any. My surgeon, though, is a careful record keeper and ordered some anyway.

When the film came back, he stood for several minutes looking at the pictures against a lighted screen.

"Well?" I finally said. "Anything you want to share with the class?"

"Huh," he said, still looking at the film. "Huh."

I got up and stood beside him. He pointed to my bone. There, in the gap that had remained vacant all this time, was the fuzzy image of something. From each end of the bone came a cloudy white form that peaked, stretching out to points that touched at the tip. Michelangelo. I let out a hoot, and would have jumped up and down if I could.

"Pretty good," agreed my surgeon with his usual reserve.

The surgery was canceled and I went home with a very precise prescription: Keep doing what you're doing.

*

It is now three years since my accident, and the bone is solid. I am sometimes asked if I think yoga cured me. Yes, it did, but not in the most obvious sense of giving me back my leg. I also had excellent surgeons and the best of Western medicine on my side. But even though Western medicine has made it possible to reattach a body part, the brain and spirit can't so easily reintegrate that which has been made separate. Yogi Bhajan, spiritual leader of the Sikhs and the man who is credited with bringing Kundalini yoga to the West, once said that yoga is the "inner science of the self." This science doesn't give you anything you don't already have. It simply provides a way to experience the wholeness of what and who you really are.

I walk with a slight limp that tends to get worse when I'm tired. I indeed cannot run, but I can dance, and I do ride, five days a week, and while I still can't achieve some asanas, neither can half the class. Everyday, each of us just has to begin where we are.

the meaning of brahmacharya
Adrian M. S. Piper

"It doesn't have to mean literally no sex whatsoever."
"It's simply not appropriate for this culture."
"Besides, most of those so-called 'renunciates' are just horny old men."
"Yeah, social losers."

Brahmacharya–translated as "celibacy" by authoritative San-skrit dictionaries–is a difficult topic to discuss in the Western yoga community. Sensory stimulation, consumption, and grati-fication are too central to contemporary Western culture to leave any of us untouched, and Freudian psychology tells us we are sexually abnormal if we are. In the yoga community, this pre-sents a further dilemma: Almost all of the ancient Vedantic and Yogic texts recommend brahmacharya for the serious yoga prac-titioner. But Indian gurus often conclude, upon their arrival in

I am grateful to Norman Bryson, Raphael Gunner, Julie Matthaei, Chuck Miller, and Lois Nesbitt for comments on earlier drafts, and to Valerie Jeremijenko for editorial help.

this culture, that this recommendation is almost impossible for their Westernized disciples to follow. Many of those who do follow it experience it as a form of unjustified deprivation that proves ultimately unpalatable. And most of those Indian gurus themselves, after extended immersion in Western culture, become vulnerable to its enticements and values to the extent of violating or renouncing this prescription in their own behavior.

This situation engenders a pervasive sense of internal conflict when the question of brahmacharya is raised. Pressured by ancient scriptures to practice it and by contemporary Western culture to reject it, yoga practitioners feel either guilty within the yoga community for violating the injunctions of the Yoga Sutra, or socially punished outside it for violating a Western standard of psychological normalcy. Conversations about sadhana inevitably turn to the value of brahmacharya, and usually the judgment is negative, if not downright disparaging. Those who identify themselves as brahmacharins often receive alternating blasts of respect, pity, and animosity within the yoga community and, outside it, incomprehension, hostility, or the insinuation that one must have a social disease.

I have practiced hatha, raja, jnana, and karma yoga since 1965; and brahmacharya since 1985. So I speak from experience of these conflicting hostile reactions. I remember how exhilarated I felt when I first discovered what it meant concretely to practice brahmacharya as a serious spiritual discipline. Indulging as usual my impulse to proselytize about my latest enthusiasm, I attempted to share this discovery with longstanding friends. Most of my male friends stampeded to the exits, while so many of my women friends engaged me in heated arguments—shouting matches, actually—that calling a truce of silence on this topic became the only way to preserve civilized discourse on any other. Within the yoga community, with few exceptions, communications tended to shut down more quickly, before the stampede or shouting stage had been reached. After these experiences I became more cautious, and revealed my commitment only when I sensed sympathy and interest, similar values and aspirations, or an incipient amorous advance.

37

The circumstances that engendered this essay—and my decision to publish it—were the quintessential last straw. I was in a reading group on Patanjali's Yoga Sutra, among kind, thoughtful, intelligent people whom I had just met. It was my second visit to the group, and I had taken to it, and them, right away. The topic was the ethical practices—called the yamas and the niyamas—required of a serious student of yoga. Brahmacharya is one of those requirements, and the usual barrage of disparaging comments began.

My stomach began to sink, and I recognized a dilemma familiar from a very different situation, in which I am in all-white company and mistaken for white; and others, not realizing I am African American, proceed to make disparaging remarks about African Americans in my presence.

The difference was that in those situations, disparaging remarks about African Americans mark my companions as unattractive company with whom I instantly lose any further desire to socialize. So I lose nothing by revealing my identity and thereby alienating them. In this situation, by contrast, disparaging remarks about brahmacharya marked my companions merely as in need of more information about it. So I stood to lose a great deal, whether I remained silent and so deceived them; or revealed myself and so alienated them. In the end it felt more important to establish relationships of integrity and trust with them than to avoid their ire or its possible consequences. So after overcoming several failures of nerve, I took the risk and "came out" as a brahmacharin. Their friendly and respectful responses were not at all what I had expected from past experience. They gave me the resolve to raise the general level of discussion of this issue so I that I would never find myself in such a predicament again.

My yoga practice itself, and particularly my meditation practice, has helped me to do this. In yogic meditation (samyama), one aim is to be able to regard the attributes and experiences of the individual ego-self from the perspective of a transpersonal witness-consciousness (or atman in Vedanta, the philosophical view that, together with yogic practice, is first described in the

Upanishads). This perspective has many benefits—among them a sense of detached amusement and compassion about one's own flaws and failures, and a keener and more pervasive sense of the tragicomic aspects of the human condition. It is also extremely useful in approaching and using for expressive or didactic purposes certain subject matter that others might regard as overly personal or private—specifically that which concerns race or gender identity. One result of my meditation practice is that those attributes do not seem all that personal or private to me. To me they are relatively superficial and generalized aspects of my external self-presentation that do not define at a deep level the person I am. Since I do not, for the most part, feel deeply attached to or invested in those particulars of my own condition, I do not feel I reveal anything particularly novel or illuminating by interrogating them as objects of public scrutiny (novelty and illumination both being, of course, relative to one's preconceptions. In fact, in order to forestall a particularly likely subset of preconceptions, let me state up front that the policy governing self-stimulation for brahmacharins is: Hands above the sheets!).

The head-on conflict of cultural values—between the East and the West, the yoga community and the Westernized secular community, brahmacharins and nonbrahmacharins—creates a fertile breeding ground for rationalization among those of us who, as deeply indoctrinated products of Western values, nevertheless respect Eastern values, and so try sincerely in our own lives to reconcile the conflict between them. The form these rationalizations usually take is to question what the term *brahmacharya* really means. To be sure, its authoritative Sanskrit translation as "celibacy" is generally acknowledged. But sometimes the terms *celibacy* and *continence* are used interchangeably. Since continence can also mean "strength," or "self-control," can't brahmacharya also mean merely "sexual self-control"? If it can, then can't one practice brahmacharya while being sexually active, as long as one is not too active, or uncontrollably active? This reasoning leads many to conclude that what brahmacharya really means is sex with only one person, i.e., monogamy; or sex only for purposes of procreation; or sex only at certain times of the

month; or sex without orgasm; or "personal energy manage-
ment" more generally, including but not limited to sexual
energy; or abstention from sex for a limited period of time in
order to enhance sex over the long term. Through such reasoning the original and clear meaning of the term *brahmacharya* is
obscured and transformed into its exact opposite.

Another variation on this reasoning focuses on the literal
meaning of the term, which is "walking with God." What does
walking with God have to do with celibacy? Can't one walk with
God by strictly observing all the *other* yamas and niyamas Patanjali enumerates? So that brahmacharya ends up having nothing
to do with celibacy at all, but rather with attaining a state of god-
liness through the practice of restraints and observances less
inimical to Western values?

The answer to all of these wistful questions is no. Brahmacharya means what the dictionaries say it means, and not something easier or more appealing for us to accept. It means something that is difficult for us to accept because it describes a
practice that is directly antithetical to some of our most deeply
held Western values and beliefs—about health, happiness, normalcy, the good life. This is why Westernized culture relegates
brahmacharya to the monastic context. There it is acceptable
because it is seen as creating an alternative and marginalized
lifestyle that neither competes with—nor, therefore, threatens—
the Westernized secular one.

But neither the ancient Vedantic and Yogic scriptures nor
twentieth-century Indian gurus prescribe, explicitly recommend, or often even mention monasticism as a necessary condition for the practice of brahmacharya. Rather, they treat brahmacharya as one discipline among others that also include such
practices as truth telling, nonviolence, and absence of envy and
greed—all of which the yogic aspirant is enjoined to make part
of her character. So the injunction to practice brahmacharya
requires us to make a choice: either to affirm certain of our
deeply instilled Western values and simply reject this one yogic
prescription as incompatible with the lives we want for ourselves; or else to reexamine and revise those values in order to
make room for it. Either alternative is honorable; to avoid the

choice through rationalization is to remain deliberately in a state of avidya (ignorance).

The second alternative is harder. Ancient texts as well as modern writers who mean to defend the traditional practice of brahmacharya usually cite its objective benefits: health, vigor, youthfulness, the eradication of zits; the transmutation of sexual energy into spiritual energy; an acceleration of the process by which Kundalini energy is drawn up the chakras to the sahasrara chakra and samadhi thereby achieved. All of these benefits are real. But to the interested bystander they are very abstract, and external to the day-to-day, subjective experience of practicing brahmacharya. Nor do they explain what celibacy has to do with "walking with God." In fact the association between celibacy and "walking with God" alludes to the deep reasons for practicing yoga in the first place.

The year brahmacharya chose me, I was having a very bad time with the men in my life. My father had died, my marriage was collapsing, and I had just been fired after years of harassment by my male colleagues. These may seem to be extremely unpromising circumstances for making a commitment to brahmacharya: How can one be sure that such a commitment is not merely sour grapes, misanthropy, or a reaction-formation to rejection? Such concerns often go along with a belief that a commitment to brahmacharya must be an act of will, undertaken in a cool, reflective, and emotionally tranquil moment, as the result of extended mental deliberation—that is, that such a commitment is valid only if it is the outcome of an *intellectual* process. But consider the voice of the Brihadaranyaka Upanishad:

> "When a man has realized the Self, the pure, the immortal, the blissful, what craving can be left in him that he should take to himself another body, full of suffering, to satisfy it?"

Or Patanjali's remarks about the effects on brahmacharya (one of the yamas) of steadfastly practicing purity (one of the niyamas):

> "Through purity, one gains detachment from the body and aversion to physical intercourse" (Yoga Sutra II.40).

Both writers are describing not an act of intellectual deliberation or assertion of will, but rather an attitude that develops naturally, as the result of previous spiritual practice and development.

One implication is that a commitment to brahmacharya can be the result of spiritual growth rather than a precondition for it. Previous spiritual practices may dispose one to regard brahmacharya as a gift and a blessing rather than a rigor or a duty that one must undertake for the sake of further spiritual development. A further implication is that brahmacharya can involve an attitudinal transformation rather than a conscious decision or vow. Someone who is ready to practice brahmacharya may not need to exercise an act of will or deliberation. Instead he may simply follow the lead of his inclinations, and do what feels most natural and comfortable, given his attitudes at that time. The first writer describes this attitudinal transformation as the result of achieving samadhi; the second, as the result of successfully practicing the niyamas.

But is a successful spiritual practice all that is necessary? Not according to the Bhagavad Gita:

> When one dwells on the pleasures of sense, attraction for them arises in one. From attraction arises desire, the lust of possession, and this leads to passion, to anger.
>
> From passion comes mental confusion, absent-mindedness, the forgetting of duty. From this loss comes the ruin of reason, and the ruin of reason leads one to destruction.
>
> But the soul that moves in the world of the senses and yet keeps the senses in harmony, free from attraction and aversion, finds rest in quietness (II.62–64).

The writer of these verses describes causal connections among empirical events: Obsession with sensory pleasure causes attraction to it, which in turn causes lust and the desire to possess, which in turn causes passion, and so on. This is not the voice of armchair a priori reasoning, or even sudden revelation, but rather of experience. It presupposes worldly knowledge, expresses personal familiarity with the vicissitudes of life in the world of the senses, and counsels us on its pitfalls. This is the kind of insight into experience, born of experience, that we recognize as wisdom rather than mere cleverness or intelligence.

But we don't have to–indeed, we should not–take this writer's word for it. We can try it ourselves, and gain knowledge of the workings of the world firsthand. *We need that worldly knowledge in order to fully appreciate the wisdom the ancient texts offer us.* Without it, these texts are just words–inspiring ones, to be sure; but without the depth and complexity of meaning that only experience and reflection on experience can give. With it, however, these words acquire multiple meaning and application to many different areas of our lives: our attitudes toward money, work, and consumption; to food, fitness and self-image; to sex, romance, and relationships–to name just a few. These verses from the Bhagavad Gita offer us the opportunity to take a different perspective on our worldly disappointments–our recent bankruptcy or thwarted career ambitions, our weight "problems" or addiction to alcohol, tobacco, or M&Ms; our recent divorce, string of failed relationships, or "intimacy problems"–again, to name just a few. These verses offer the possibility of thinking of these disappointments as revelatory of certain internal causal mechanics of the world of sensory gratification.

However, our attachment to this world, and to the Western standards of power, achievement, acquisition, health, beauty, or personal charisma that govern and reinforce it, usually leads us to the opposite conclusion. Such disappointments are viewed as revelatory, not of the workings of the world, but rather of our personal failure to live up to its requirements. We may conclude that we have an addiction to shopping, or lack self-control over food, or are too deficient in social skills to maintain a satisfying sexual relationship. We then–if we have a healthy sense of self-esteem–find the relevant repair shop, pick ourselves up, dust ourselves off, and resume the pursuit of sensory gratification with renewed optimism that next time we will get it (whatever "it" is) right.

By contrast, the ethics of the Vedic *Brahmanas* regards this pursuit differently. It stipulates four different ends or ideals of life (purusharthas). Each of these is appropriate to a different period in a person's life, and its pursuit guides the lifestyle and practices appropriate to that period. Wealth (artha) is the goal of the first twenty-five years of one's life, brahmacharya ashrama. This period is devoted to learning and training, in order to make one's way in the world and to achieve economic well-being. During this period celibacy is a means to maintaining one's focus on study. Desire-satisfaction (kama) is the goal of the second twenty-five years of one's life, grihastha ashrama. During this period, one seeks and finds a mate, begets a family, and becomes a householder, utilizing one's economic wealth for the well-being of oneself and one's relations. Around the age of fifty, in the period of vanaprastha ashrama, one begins to question one's lifestyle and achievements and to search for deeper meaning in one's life. Ethical values, character, and guidance (dharma) become more important than worldly success or desire-satisfaction, and one develops an interest in meditation and study of the scriptures. One begins to retire from the world of profit and gratification, and gradually to shed its trappings. Around the age of seventy-five, the sanyasa ashrama stage, one has fully experienced worldly success and the vicissitudes of the world of sensory gratification, and has reflected on and revised one's order of priorities toward the ethical and spiritual. One is then ready to devote the remainder of one's life to the search for union with ultimate reality (moksha), by renouncing the world of sensory gratification altogether.

Certainly these four stages of life will be less clear-cut, structured, and ritualized in the less structured and ritualized society of the West. The time periods may not divide one's life so evenly into four equal segments, so that one may spend less time, or more, in study or professional training; or less time, or more, as a grihastha or vanaprastha; or be called to the pursuit of moksha –and possibly a monastic life–at an earlier age. If one is pursuing an alternative lifestyle, or living in a vowed or intentional community, or is gay or lesbian, the formation of a household and of familial relationships may not follow the traditional Vedic model. Nor may the segmented model of education followed by worldly work conform closely to one's professional arrangements.

The importance of the concept of the four purusharthas is that it makes a valued place for the world of the senses, for the pursuit of power, success, and gratification. It acknowledges and legitimizes the natural human urges we all have to engage with this world, to seek our paths in it, and to cull from it the experience, worldly knowledge, and finally the wisdom it has to offer. It acknowledges the importance and value of full engagement with the world, *and* it adds that to get stuck at this particular stage of human growth is a case of arrested development. It tells us that at a certain point, we are *supposed* to give up our ascetic devotion to our studies and plunge into the world of desire and ambition; that at a later point, we are *supposed* to become disenchanted with that world and seek beyond it for something more meaningful; and that we are then *supposed* to find and embrace what we are ultimately looking for with such love and fervor that there is then nothing to do but get rid of all the impediments to devoting oneself wholeheartedly to the journey that leads beyond death.

This alternative ethical tradition creates potent possibilities for revising one's judgments about circumstances and relationships that would count as failed or abnormal according to Western standards. Take, for example, a longstanding intimate relationship in which sex no longer occurs, or no longer satisfies; or a series of relationships seemingly thwarted by sexual needs; or the desire for a relationship in which the expectation of sex appears to be an insurmountable barrier; or the longing for a genuine meeting of minds beyond the complications of sexual involvement; or for solitude. Maybe these interpersonal conditions have nothing to do with anyone's failings or inadequacies or pathologies. Maybe they are signals that it is time to explore other options within oneself or the relationship. That is, maybe these interpersonal conditions are opportunities to be investigated, rather than catastrophes to be ameliorated as quickly as possible.

Indeed, the Vedic ethical tradition offers the possibility of turning our entire system of relationship priorities inside out. Maybe the real point of a relationship between two people is spiritual rather than sexual union. Maybe we should seek spiritual rather than sexual compatibility in a partner, and regard sex as an afterthought, on a par with hobbies such as stamp collecting. Maybe sexual attraction is merely a decoy, a distraction that depends on rather than transcends boundaries between individuals. Maybe sexual passion is a transient phase—we might call it the Rabbit Phase—that two people really must just endure and suffer through. Maybe the right response to sexual attraction is to just grit one's teeth and ride it out (so to speak), so that one can then move beyond it to the really important part of the relationship: the union of mind and spirit that no physical or temporal boundaries can contain. To move through and beyond the world of the senses is to put that world to the use for which it is meant: to deepen our insight into the nature of ultimate reality, and prepare ourselves for final union with it. This is part of the insight that the preceding verses of the Bhagavad Gita attempt to communicate to us. The only question is whether we are at the stage of being able fully to receive it.

When I first read the above verses from the Bhagavad Gita in the mid-1960s, I was not ready to receive their insights—at least not consciously. I was too young and frisky. I felt a strong need to go mix it up in the world of maya, and so that is what I did for a couple of decades. It was a good party. During my Bad Year With Men I did not draw any of the inferences described earlier, and I did not feel ready at all to move on to another stage. Instead I took my newfound circumstances as a jobless and fatherless divorcée as a comment on my flawed personal and professional skills, rather than on the course of the world; and was desperate to get it right the next time. My relationship antennae were up and circling in all directions, searching far and wide for a new partner to give me the love, support, and protection I felt I needed.

Oddly enough, every time a likely suitor appeared on the horizon, I skittered away. After this had happened a number of times (I am a very slow learner in these matters), it finally dawned on me that my actions and bodily reactions were trying to tell me something that I needed to heed: to back off for a while, and relax. So I did that. I withdrew my antennae, indeed withdrew from my sexuality altogether, and watched, and wrote, and read, and analyzed, and processed all that I had been through. I became invisible to the opposite sex, and watched the sexualized messages, fashions, advertising, entertainment, peer pressure, habits, relationships, and interactions all around me, filtering everything through the lens of my experiences, my reading, and my daily journal writing.

During this time I had been functionally celibate for three years—the first time since the age of eleven that I had been without a mate in my life for more than a few months. My sadhana, practiced daily on my own since 1972, had deepened. It consisted of a homegrown, hour-long vinyasa coordinated by ujjayi and kapalabhati, followed by about an hour of advanced pranayama and an hour of meditation. I have also been a vegetarian since 1967, nicotine free since 1968, caffeine free since 1974, and alcohol and weed free since 1988. Since 1968 I have tried to conduct a twenty-four-hour water fast one day a week, although I don't always succeed. I confess to mild addictions to *People* magazine and *Star Trek*. I mention all of these habits because I believe they have some bearing on what occurred one day during meditation, within a week of embarking on a conscious tentative commitment to brahmacharya.

What occurred was a very gentle and gradual opening and deepening. My sensory experience became sharper, more vivid, intricate, and singular; my peripheral vision broader and more encompassing. My visual field and everything in it grew vast, timeless, and very, very clear. Everything and everyone had a familiarity and intimacy, and at the same time great mystery, dignity, and breathtaking majesty. The world radiated a magisterial stillness behind the noise and sounds of daily urban life. Those sounds themselves had a sweetness and magic beneath their mundane meanings. All of it filled my mind and my senses so completely that I as an experiencing subject disappeared from the picture. My bodily habits regarding nourishment, sleep, and so on receded into the background, until they became needs that sharply signaled their presence and demanded attention. Satis-fying them had the same texture as the rest of this experience, only not as interesting.

At the same time that my cognition and perception of my sur-roundings were expanding, my inner space—my mental interior, which I experience as the area approximately from the inside of the head to the throat to the abdomen—opened onto the boundless universe of deep space. Kinesthetically, there was no "place" where "I" was "sitting" "upright," because all those spatial indices of location and orientation ceased to exist. My movement through my environment was nevertheless light, effortless, and sure. What did exist was the vast expanse of the universe, and its ancient echo-hum. It was too deep and low and penetrating to be a sound (although it can be replicated at the level of sound by chanting "OM"), too pervasive to divide objects and things from one another, but pervasive enough to imbue all of my percep-tions—of my visual field, the objects and people in it, my body and its environment—with its vibration. The clarity, intricacy, and vibrational depth of each person and thing made each an object of fascination, astonishment, and unique and inestimable value. Everything revealed its timeless and limitless splendor simulta-neously. As a whole, the experience was comparable to psyche-delically induced ones I'd had in the sixties; less profoundly transformative, but also gentler and less invasive. It lasted for about a week, until I shut myself down.

I shut myself down because local circumstances and a gener-ally inhospitable lifestyle demanded more armor and less vul-nerability than this experience induced in me. In my ordinary life I have to be a warrior on many fronts: racial, social, gender, academic (I was the only tenured black woman in philosophy—a field that numbers about 15,000—until 1994), artistic (I make difficult, confrontational art about racism that gets me into trou-ble with most people). Because yogic scriptures tend to come from the Brahminic caste, the prescriptions and recommenda-tions ordinarily found in texts on karma yoga tend to often pre-suppose a basically benevolent environment, in which the main issue is how one can maintain serenity in the face of adversity

and virtue in the face of temptation. Often they counsel the culti-
vation of detachment, love, and compassion—for oneself as well
as for others. I call it the sweetness-and-light approach. These
presuppositions and recommendations are largely compatible
with those of the white, upper-middle-class audience yoga tends
to find in the West. They tend not to address squarely the problem
of evil, i.e., how one should respond to acts of malice, cruelty,
sadism, brutality, or annihilation directed against oneself by
individuals for whom one's very existence is an insult to be erad-
icated as quickly and effectively as possible.

49

I have found the traditional counsel useful only to a certain
extent. More useful, in my experience, are particular yamas and
niyamas to which I find I am particularly attracted, in my artistic
and philosophical work as well as in my life. My commitment to
jnana yoga makes satya—translated as "truth" and more generally as "the avoidance of falsehood"—very personally important
to me; as it does svadhyaya (self-study). Satya means seeking and
speaking the truth, and also refusing to collude in falsehood. It
means refusing to support both one's own self-deceptions—here
it becomes svadhyaya—and the self-deceptions and social delu-
sions of others, even when they are deeply instilled by cultural
and environmental forces. I regard satya as a freely available
weapon for fighting ignorance, dishonesty, and disingenu-
ousness—and the dangerous actions guided by them—by speaking or otherwise expressing the truth, even though this may be
troubling or painful to the speaker as well as to the listener.
(Thus satya, in my opinion, overrides ahimsa [nonviolence] in
some circumstances.) The only way I have ever found to survive
lethal assaults on my person or spirit is to make use of this
weapon to the best of my ability; to get my dukes up, protect my
back, and come out swinging. That is what I did.

Since then I have kept up the personal practices I described
earlier. My asana practice has been influenced by my reentry, in
1992, to the world of hatha yoga classes—which had undergone a
profound transformation during the twenty years I was away
from them. Because my original meditation experience was so
opening and enveloping, so inspiring of awe and reverence,

bhakti yogic practices—kirtan, japam, ishta-deva pranam—have assumed a larger role in my sadhana. These, in turn, have deepened my meditation practice even more, and increased my access to that experience. The easier it gets to blast off, the more I have restricted for now my pranayama practice, in anticipation of the time when I will be free to blast off as far and fast as I like.

Some things have remained the same. If I duplicate all of the yogic practices I was doing then, I can replicate the experience I had then. I have done that several times, and more recently by simply calling it forth, without duplicating the practices. Once it occurred while I was chanting the Bija Mantra at a yoga retreat. I am constantly reminded of the nearness of that world by the sharpness and vividness of detail I still perceive in inanimate objects, and the singular and unique personalities I still find in all sentient things (yes, I talk to plants. I even talk to cockroaches before I, um, liberate them). I live with the awareness that the world received in that way is there, very close at hand, waiting for me, whenever I am ready. I am in the process of getting ready, and am very protective of my access to it. I remember what it was like to have effectively forgotten what reality is really like, to have lost the immanent presence of that world in a fog of personal and social preoccupations, desires, and ambitions; to have operated on the practical assumption that those mundane and worldly concerns were all there were, and to have effectively lost all clue about what lay beyond the surface appearances of things. I remember what it was like to give lip service to the existence and importance of that deeper reality without concretely experiencing it. I don't want to get lost in the world of maya ever again.

As the result of my meditation experience, my perceptual appreciation of physical beauty, fineness of sensibility, and depth of spirit in others has been greatly enhanced; and the search for kindred spirits, who know what I know and have been where I have been, has become much more urgent. I have also gained tremendous respect for the power of sexuality as a natural biological force that can create or annihilate anything—conventions, restraints, inhibitions, individuals, relationships, families, reputations, livelihoods, lives—that stands in its way. I feel nothing but gratitude and relief that it seems to have gotten out of mine. I do not believe in free will in general, and I have never thought that individuals have very much control over the effect of biological forces on their sexual behavior. When I look back on my own it seems to me a miracle that I am still alive to allude to it.

Moreover, the hatha sadhana I now practice—an Ashtanga-style vinyasa grounded in the formal techniques and structural approach of Iyengar yoga—presents a particular challenge to my commitment to brahmacharya. Ashtanga yoga is an intensely, unapologetically spiritual practice. From the first moments in a led class, the beginner is confronted by having to stand with her hands in prayer position, and chant "OM" and a lengthy Sanskrit invocation. Thereafter the coordination of asana, ujjayi breathing, control of internal muscles (the bandhas) and meditative focus of the gaze (the drishtis) is emphasized. This practice calls on all aspects of awareness simultaneously, and arouses an intensely meditative and devotional state. Unlike Iyengar, Bikram, or power yoga (to name just a few alternative styles), it is not possible to practice this type of hatha yoga without coming into immediate contact with its sacred dimension.

On the other hand, Ashtanga has another dimension that can easily become profane under certain circumstances. Because Ashtanga yoga coordinates the simultaneous development of strength and flexibility, there comes a point in the development of strength when developing further flexibility requires the teacher to give the student assists that are not only hands-on, but in many cases body-on. In baddha konasana, for example, the teacher might kneel behind the student, his knees on her upper thighs and hands on her knees, and gradually lower the full weight of his torso and chest onto the entire length of her back, simultaneously opening her groin and lengthening her back as she bends forward while lifting her heart. The physical intimacy of these assists can express a chaste, caring, and respectful relationship between student and teacher. It can also be a Really Fast Way to Get Babes (female or male). It is not always a simple matter—either for teacher or for student—to distinguish between these two attitudes. A commitment to brahmacharya may arouse conflicts between the sacred and the profane that are not easy for either teacher or student to resolve. Simply announcing this commitment does not necessarily resolve the conflict, and may even exacerbate it.

So I would never rule out the possibility that I might, despite what I have found, revert to Rabbit Phase nevertheless. But since then I have been seriously tempted only once. The situation was prohibitive enough, and the potential costs high enough, to be adequately discouraging; he then cooperated by behaving badly (although not badly enough to make it easy). Moreover, the quality of the friendships I have formed, selectively, with the opposite sex would be very hard to relinquish. For it turns out that those of my former male friends who beat a hasty retreat when I revealed my commitment to brahmacharya were the ones who needed to think of me as sexually available to them, even if only in theory, as a condition of interacting with me at all. They were the majority. But others (a very small minority) who were secure enough in their gender identities to explore more advanced dimensions of relationship with women reacted by relaxing their defenses, knowing that I would not make sexual demands on them. Their acceptance of me despite my commitment enabled me to relax my defenses, secure in the knowledge that they would make no such demands on me. With lowered defenses on both sides has come increased vulnerability, increased trust, increased intimacy, increased freedom of self-expression. The result has been that my friendships with men, though *many* fewer in number, tend to be deeper and more respectful than before. It is difficult to avoid the conclusion that these improvements depend on observing the constraints brahmacharya demands.

An increasingly popular, Westernized version of Hinduism's Tantric tradition claims that one can have it both ways: both sex and samadhi together, as it were. I am not convinced. Tantra developed around 500 C.E. out of the ancient polytheistic culture of the Indian subcontinent. This culture predates the Aryan settlement of the Indus Valley around 3000 B.C.E. The Aryan-composed Vedas, the most ancient religious and philosophical scriptures in the world, include the Upanishads, cornerstone of

Advaita Vedanta–an orthodox, nondualistic philosophy contingently associated with the Brahmin priests of Hinduism. What has been humorously referred to as "California Tantra" is fundamentally in conflict with Advaita Vedanta.

Tantra developed in many directions. Some directions emphasize worship of the divine mother, or complex meditational visualization, rather than sexual rites or practices. Tantra is also often described as the "left-handed path" contingently associated with the lower castes, women, and outcasts. In some Tantric cults, the habits and actions conceived by the priests as obstacles to liberation–carnivorism, sex, intoxication, blood sacrifice, transgression of established social norms and rituals–are used instead as means to it. The basic idea is that liberation from the constraints of the individual ego-self can be achieved by imitating the amorality of the gods and performing certain rites and rituals that identify one with them. The practice that has engendered most interest in the West emphasizes the achievement of ecstatic self-transcendence through sexual acts and rites in which the participants imitate and identify with, for example, Siva and Shakti, the god and goddess of destruction and creative power respectively.

In Advaita Vedanta, Siva, Shakti, and other traditional Hindu deities are assimilated and reconceived as divine personifications of a nondual, unified first cause known as Brahman that precedes and generates the world of multiplicity and natural forces. This first cause is an all pervasive *state* of conscious intelligence, rather than a discriminable *entity*. In traditional Tantra, by contrast, Siva and Shakti are two of many such deities, each of which has its role, function, and personality in social and religious life, and each of which demands its own form of supplication. And in Kashmir Shaivism, the most sophisticated expression of Hindu Tantra, even that first cause itself, the god Siva with whom we are to identify, is particularized as a deity–and therefore as a discriminable *entity*–by the attributes of will, freedom, intention, omnipotence–much as in Judeo-Christian monotheism.

My biggest (but not my only) complaint about California Tantra is the inadequacy of its conception of self-transcendence, which decouples the experience of liberation from the experience of illumination. Illumination is a *cognitive* experience of insight into the ultimate nature of reality that finds no place in California Tantra. To see this, compare California Tantra, Western philosophy, and Advaita Vedanta. One of the most interesting differences between Western philosophy and science on the one hand and Advaita Vedanta on the other is in their respective epistemologies. Western philosophy and science conceive our access to ultimate reality as propositional, i.e., as encoded in universal, explanatory first principles that denote a level of reality that is experientially inaccessible to us. So when and if we succeed in formulating such principles correctly, we will have only an intellectual understanding of that reality. We arrive at the formulation of these final principles through techniques of empirical observation and experimentation, inductive and deductive reasoning, and theory construction.

In Advaita Vedanta, by contrast, epistemic access to ultimate reality is through direct experience, unmediated by extrinsic processes, techniques, or conceptualization. Instead this direct access is achieved with the aid of the mental and physical disciplines of yoga, which modify and strengthen the mind, body, and central nervous system so as to comprehend and process this experience safely. Thus insight is the fruit of revelation rather than of reasoning. Because it involves an unmediated relationship between the knowing subject and the object known, the subjective distinction between them is effectively erased. So the experience of direct access to ultimate reality is an experience of union with it; and transcending the constraints of the individual ego-self and fully grasping the universal first principles that govern ultimate reality are one and the same. Because Advaita Vedantic epistemology requires the full involvement of the person as a necessary condition of obtaining ultimate knowledge (or, more properly speaking, wisdom), it is much more demanding of all of one's capacities than Western epistemology, which exercises only the intellect. On the Advaita Vedantic view, self-transcendence–liberation–consists in a certain kind of insight; namely, in an unmediated experience of and union with ultimate reality.

California Tantra, by contrast, promises self-transcendence through–well, sex, drugs, and rock 'n' roll. And hamburgers, and also Coke. And maybe M&Ms. It delivers on this promise insofar as certain sexual practices, intoxicants, and rituals of rhythmic dance and movement facilitate the experience of temporarily freeing oneself from one's limiting attitudes, inhibitions, and customary behavior. This degree and quality of liberation is real, and nothing to sneeze at. What it does not do, even under the most serious and well-intentioned of circumstances, even when all ritual prescriptions are carefully observed, is lead one beyond identification with the god or goddess of one's choice to a deeper cognitive experience of insight into the first principles that structure the universe in which that god or goddess has a place. Because California Tantra derives its motivation and cosmology from a basically polytheistic worldview, its conception of self-transcendence stops short of finally transcending the world of ·multiplicity in an act of cognitive union. Advaita Vedanta can be understood as the median between the extremes of Western epistemology, which engages only the intellect, and California Tantra, which engages the mind and senses but has no proper epistemology at all. Compared to the experience of direct and unmediated union with ultimate reality on which Advaita Vedanta is premised, the California Tantric experience of mere sexual union between cosmic divinities does not convince me that one can have both sex and samadhi together.

Central to my meditation experience was the way my bodily needs and desires receded proportionally into the background and then disappeared, as I let the world as it really is into my self more and more completely. It felt natural and easy then, and it does now, too. Very often so-called ascetic practices are conceived in the spirit of renunciation and self-deprivation–of food, sex, alcohol, drugs, tobacco, partying, M&Ms; as though the point of the practice is self-flagellation or the assertion of will; and as though by breaking our attachment to these things we end up with less rather than more. I think this is a mistake; and that if one feels deprived by their lack one should have as much food, sex, M&Ms, etc. as one needs in order to feel deprived instead by their surfeit. Variants on a general rule of thumb might be: Party until you've gotten your yayas out; or until you've had enough partying for three lifetimes; or until you've learned the lessons from it you need to learn.

The point of "ascetic" practices is not what one gives up but rather what one gets. Giving up M&Ms and so forth is a negligible price to pay. The point is to *get one's self, one's needs, one's desires, and one's preoccupations out of the way,* so that the universe can drop more deeply into one's consciousness for a visit; so that other people—all other people, not just the current object of one's affection—can be seen and sensed and received more clearly, and their singular mystery and depth comprehended and felt and valued more directly; so that objects and environments and events can make their unique and imperturbable presences felt more intensely, all along one's surfaces and beyond them; so that all of it can inhabit one vividly, simultaneously, and timelessly.

Recently I was trying to make this point to a Tantric Buddhist friend of mine. Itching for a fight, he commented, "So, basically, Adrian, what you're saying is that you give up the good life so you can get fucked by the universe?"

Ahem. Well, not quite. One does not give up the good life, but rather maximizes its goodness. As to one's relationship with the universe, to design one's life and one's sadhana so as to make it easy for the universe not only to drop in for a visit, but to take up permanent residence in one's body and mind is what it means to "walk with God."

lyric yoga
Stanley Plumly

1

I blame, in part, my sometimes inability to sit still on those hours of hardwood silence endured at meeting. They felt unendurable, I'm sure, because, at nine or ten or twelve years of age, sitting still for long stretches is antithetical to a child's nature and because breaking the silence by speaking in front of a lot of people, especially people as alternately dour or fired up as Quakers, is worse. Even the adults, I remember thinking, must be speaking up in order to relieve the body's boredom. I don't believe that by college meeting got more comfortable—not that comfort was its point—so

I finally stopped going and ultimately chose to meditate and articulate by other means: in solitude and at the typewriter.

What I took away from Quaker collective meditation was the good sense of stillness–not so much its length in time as its presence within the space of things, which translated as the need for reflection, a sense of order and mindfulness, and as a way to reach the insights of contemplation, the deep interior moment. The Quaker concept of the inner light became an opportunity for self-interrogation, self-witness. Giving witness, I later remembered, was exactly what meeting was all about. And stillness and its silence were the place where you could arrive at an understanding of mind and heart, even if you kept it to yourself.

Stillness within the self, within the silence. Being alone is what writing is about. Writing is giving witness. In my attention-deficit years, sitting in meeting in relative motionlessness inside a cave of Quaker rectitude was difficult enough; the thought of having to stand–worse than in school–and speak from whatever shallow depths of my being I could muster was paralyzing. My tongue turned to wood, hardwood. When I started, seriously, to write I learned that being alone with blank white paper was no less intimidating, no less a publicity. I also learned that stillness was inwardness and a way to prepare to speak, the dream and daydream the content of the words. Writing became the restlessness answering the stillness. To the degree that sitting still, moving inward, having insight are virtues of meditative silence, the complexity of the process also involves finding a form to express the experience. Poetry, for me, was that form.

2

Stillness and restlessness, related or separate, have become one of my poetry's themes. More importantly, they have become essential to the way I make poems, the way I sit in a chair and address the page and the way I interrupt myself to pace or think or empty the moment in order to start again. Writing–its concentrations, demands, anxieties, joys, backs and forths–is so intimately tied to the body and at the same time about leaving the body that it's sometimes impossible to distinguish into twos its singular experience. which is why most writers' time at the desk means getting lost in time. The physical body becomes the host for the spiritual traveler. In this sense, stillness comes to represent the body, restlessness the imagination.

One, however, could easily argue the matter the other way around. That is the beauty of polarity. Restlessness *is* the body's inclination, stillness the spirit's great desire, not unlike T. S. Eliot's famous Chinese jar moving perpetually in its stillness. The body sits at its angle of repose or angst and allows the mind to do its work, just as the fingers translate, even transform, what the mind speaks. Are the words on the field of the page more physical or spiritual realities, actual or ontological, or is one merely passage to the other, not possible without the other–in effect, a simultaneity? This is, of course, a rhetorical question. We are told, in various philosophies, that the alphabetical letters I'm writing right now simultaneously stand for something, like agreeable math. But if the letters are obscure, the handwriting poor, the typing sloppy, the words on the computer screen ungrammatical, the sentences in makeshift paragraphs confusing, what is represented except an attempt at communication? Writing, literally, needs to be artistic; writing, figuratively, must be art. The subtleties, the tones, the implications, the nuances, the edges and angles, meanings and possibilities are otherwise blurred, distorted, dumb.

The act of writing may be a restlessness. The result is its stillness, a text fit for both contemplation and revelation. Writing perfects the writer; it also completes longing in the reader. Writing and reading are stillness and restlessness closed into a whole performance. In "Thirteen Ways of Looking at a Blackbird," Wallace Stevens states that he doesn't know which to prefer,

> *The beauty of inflections*
> *Or the beauty of innuendoes,*
> *The blackbird whistling*
> *Or just after.*

For the writer, subsumed in the silence of making something, there's little difference between before and after, memory and the moment, the instant and its resonance. The inflection is the innuendo. The restlessness can only speak through stillness, just as the fullness must first be empty.

> *Your whole life you are two with one taken*
> *away. The inadequate air and fire,*
> *the inadequate joy, the darkness*
> *of the room so gathered at the window*
> *as to fly, wing on wing on wing open*
> *against the glass, opening and closing,*
> *bone, blood and wrist. But nothing happens but*
> *exhaustion and evidence of the eyes,*
> *the red-gold cloud-break morning beginning*
>
> *with the objects that floated in the dark*
> *draining back to the source, floating back to*
> *the surface tension of things, those objects*
> *struck the way the first light starts suddenly,*
> *then slowly in relief across the room,*
> *the window's shadow garden come back one*
> *last time once more from the leaves. Waking now,*
> *the door half-open, open, the doorway's*
> *blindness or blackness silence to be filled.*

These first two stanzas from a forty-five line poem of mine refer to a series of mornings when I'd wake up with the early light and wait, in half-sleep, for the full sun. The time seemed interminable—a throwback to the internal time of meetings in my childhood—with the graduating shadow-play of sunlight through the window a drama unto itself. Slow waking was a coming into consciousness, while the body lay in recess. Slow waking was also the mind coming alive, making connections, associations, organizing an inferred narrative. The lighter it got the richer the visual mix. When I thought about the experience later, and over the next many days and weeks, it turned into language, into an imaginative event, based on an understanding of and insight into what started it. Writing became a meditation of a meditative moment: a mediation, in fact, of what became a spiritual experience. The whistling and just after.

Everything I've so far said about stillness and poetry, about the byplay and polarity of restlessness and stillness, meditation and silence, insight and articulation can be applied to the principles and practice of yoga. This is true whether one is seeking physical or spiritual focus, epiphany or some involuntary combination, whether one is looking for holistic health or the sublimity of beatitude. To say that poetry is a kind of yoga, or the other way around, is to observe the obvious. And yoga is no less susceptible to cliché than poetry is. Yoga has become so generic an American activity and so generally applied that what one means by invoking it may be one thing here and another there. One hears of power yoga, slow yoga, aerobic yoga, movement yoga, dancing yoga; one is distantly aware of Tantra yoga, jnana yoga, raja yoga; and through a graduation of asanas or pure pranayama, one may wish to achieve a state approaching true kundalini. Yoga may be, according to *Psychology Today*, the fastest-growing "fitness training" in America, but you have to wonder what the Bhagavad Gita or the Upanishads or the Vedic hymns would make of yoga as gym art.

B. K. S. Iyengar has commented that "the original idea of yoga is freedom and beatitude, and the by-products which come along the way, including physical health, are secondary for the practitioner." Iyengar has trained many of the contemporary American teachers of hatha yoga, who themselves are now teachers. *Hatha* refers to that force within us that, when released, leads to self-transformation, self-transcendence. Yoga postures are part of the means to that end. They include siddha-asana and mountain pose, both emphatic postures of vertical stillness. It's hard to get away from the body, the form, as the vessel in which the content of the mind, heart, and spirit are lifted; it's hard to get away from the spine as the ascending ladder or the breath as the good ghost of our being. Yoga fails when the body becomes the end in itself; yet yoga is only hot air without the body to bear its message. In the short seven years I've been doing yoga, at a kind of good middling second level, I've come to realize that though performing the postures themselves may be the blackbird whistling, the real effect comes just after, when the freedom of the release becomes joy.

Writing poems may or may not be yoga by other means. Poems as such, however, do take on the dynamic interactions implicit in yoga, particularly in the way that form and content, body and mind, turn inseparable. Poems, in this sense, like all art, represent the ideas as well as the ideals of the poses: balance, breath, movement within stillness, clarity, empathy, discovery, inevitability, release, and the quiet sublime of a reference outside the self. The claims of yoga, nevertheless, are only as good as its practice, regardless of any high-minded rhetoric surrounding its teaching. The same is true for poetry, or of any human activity that aspires to grace. When I think about it, Quaker meeting, writing poems, and practicing yoga, as a chronology, have formed a link in helping to create the expressive texture in my life. The experience of the one has found fulfillment in the next–to the extent that meditation and making and "posing" have melded into a single process, in which doing one recalls the others.

We say that the body is a temple, because we know that it's nothing but mortal architecture without the self-regard of consciousness and conscience. The contemplative moment draws us to our sources; we see inside. We close our eyes, in fact, in order to see with clarity. Indeed, the imagination asks us to see with our eyes closed. So we make connections in the dark and thus we imagine what our bodies can do and be, how the breath of the spirit can come and go with perfection, how the ladder gravity of the spine can soar. Poets speak of rhythm and breath as the lifeline of the poetic line; they speak of form as the embodiment of the poem's energy, the bodying forth of its meaning and being. To expire is to breathe out, to inspire is to breathe in. To aspire is to breathe with the mind, to give purpose to the heart's rhythm. The spine is an aspiration too, since it lifts us from foundations. To imagine what the body can achieve is to invest it with awareness–to begin to make it twice alive: first as a body, then as an embodiment.

Whatever vision I aspire to in my poems, I'm basically a practical person. That is, I try to live within myself and move through the world with a certain economy: economy of speech, manner, gesture, purpose, and desire. Like many practical people, I hate waste—wasted energy, wasted words, wasted means. W. B. Yeats once defined poetry as wasted breath, but he intended his description as an economical, ironic, understated observation. From a didactic point of view, poetry is wasted breath, since it's wasted into language as lyric, as music itself is wasted into the air. The poetry of yoga wastes its breath a lot like music, since breath – its expiration, inspiration, aspiration–is exercise of the spirit. Waste and renewal, waste and renewal—every pose seems to be working to right the balance between waste and renewal, the balance between giving back to the air and taking back in from the air, as if we were rediscovering the lungs of our original nature.

The first lesson of yoga is how to build an economy of breathing, how to find the best balance between the voice in the air outside and the voice within us. When that balance is abridged or confused in some way, as it so often is in the dailiness of our lives, we seem to black out a bit, become disoriented, frustrated, depressed; we start to list or stoop and suffer a diminishment. To lift the spirit—quite literally–is to correct from imbalance to balance our breathing, to reestablish its healthy, inherent economy.

In my limited experience, I've found that the actual quality and tones of voice of the yoga instructor have a great deal to do with coming to an understanding of balanced breathing. I've been lucky in that the person I've studied with for the past seven years has one of those voices that speaks from the heart without a trace of hype or strain, someone who, without the appearance of trying, transforms the instruction into images. Yoga, I've come to realize, is almost as much about the right economy of words and imagination as it is about the best balance of breath. Of course, the words are breath, and the body the extension of the breathing. The language of the instructor becomes the student's language, part of the body's honesty with itself. And what is the voice except the pose honestly enacted?

"I saw a yogi remain in the air, several feet above the ground last night at a group meeting"–this detail from Paramahansa Yogananda's *Autobiography of a Yogi*. Levitation, real or perceived, as a true or false economy, may or may not be of value. One has one's own opinions regarding the miraculous. But levitation as an internal, emotional experience, in which the body feels as if it's rising beyond itself as it's released within a pose, levitation as a rich imaginative experience of the body's victory over gravity, is exactly what true yoga economy is about. By victory I mean balance, resistance, polarity with the ground–as even, the poet says, the invisible breath of the spirit must abide the earth. The right human voice, as much a part of nature as birdsong, is words relative to the gravity or levity of their rendering. The yoga body wants to be of that voice, at one with it.

5

The sun god Apollo is not only the god of poetry but the god of light and healing. It's good to remember this connection in respect to yoga, which seeks to repair through enlightenment. The Apollonian metaphor suggests the body in darkness needing to be brought into the health of sunshine–perhaps not so much the extreme of noon as the quieter, softer healing light of dawn and sunset, each twilights in their way. Thus the figure of Apollo more than likely suggests the body and soul in shadow needing to be brought to a place beyond ambiguity and ambivalence. What I like most about the Quakers is their belief that the light is already there, inside us, at about one candlepower, meaning that it's a meditative light of understated divinity. For the ancient Greeks and Romans–as well as the Romantic John Keats–Apollo was divine. For anyone seriously studying yoga it's understood that the self itself is part of a divinity, a natural, ecumenical divinity. Like it or not, religious orthodoxy tends to be a strong noon light pouring down on things. Divinity of the spirit is more like Emily Dickinson's "certain slant of light," at early morning and evening, part of nature.

What is especially beautiful about early and late light is how quiet it is. The dark and high noon have their own special invisible sounds. But angular light is healing, and a state of beauty we are drawn to. The third stanza of the poem I quoted earlier has a Lazarus figure locked inside the tomb of his own darkness.

> *A man was sick, a sickness unto death.*
> *All he wanted to do was lie down,*
> *Let the light pick him apart like the dust.*
> *He wrapped himself in his mind, in his own*
> *absence. He did not want to hear the rain,*
> *with its meaning, nor the moment after*
> *rain, nor the sound of Jesus weeping, nor*
> *the dreaming, which is memory, though he*
> *lay a long time cold, head against the stone.*

Morning light is a coming into wakefulness, evening light into awareness. Probably the best time to practice yoga is when the sun is breaking or setting over water, a plain, or between mountains. Most of us, though, live in cities, where buildings form the landscape. It's tempting in cities to look into mirrors rather than see through windows. But yoga, emphatically in an urban landscape, is about windows, not mirrors-high windows, above of the heaviness of noise and distraction, and closer to the sun's salutation. City or country, among buildings or trees, the poetry of yoga asks us to rise from the dark weight of the night's body or the dead weight of the day's and become alive again, to be lighter in every possible way. And to see with the insight of quiet light.

When I was a boy my father and I would drive up to Canada to fish. The lakes there are famous for their stillness and darkness, their depth and cold. Evenings, sometimes, if we'd made a good catch of pike or pickerel and had a good meal, he'd let me lie in the bottom of the boat off a long line from the shore so that I could drift a little and look at the sky, which seemed like a lake itself, large and deep and pure, with gold and silver twilight ever so slowly, ever so softly about to slip under. The enormous edges of the lake were long since in silhouette and distant, and the summer sounds barely audible, so I had this feeling of floating between the stilled buoyancy of the water and the great silence of the star-filling sky. It was a feeling of immense disappearance, or of joining something larger. Perhaps it was like that feeling we have in dreams of falling or flying, where we are taken out of ourselves, if momentarily. It was a kind of feeling children often naturally discover and one that adults often try to get back to.

the practice of paradox
Alison West

The physical practice of yoga is so deeply anchored in me now that I know it more by its occasional absence. At such times, a certain physical inertia begins to set in, causing me to marvel at the profound effect the practice has on my well-being. The practice of asanas and pranayama has provided me with a range of clear, tangible sensations, among them the voluptuous, exhilarating experience like being a "feather on the breath of God," or the simple, refreshing pleasure of good, hard work, or, on days I am not inclined to accept the discipline, a burdensome nuisance.

The brilliance of the geometric structure of the asanas and the way in which they target specific bones, muscles, organs, nerves, and more subtle systems are one of the satisfactions of the physical practice, not to mention the pleasure of knowing more about the body's complex inner workings.

Above all, yoga has forced me to contend with paradox and the ineffable. Paradox would have been hard to miss or ignore and I might well have developed a preoccupation with it in another context. But as far as I can tell it was indeed yoga that encouraged this awkward interest. Ever since learning, as a schoolgirl, Blake's "To see the world in a grain of sand / And a heaven in a wildflower / Hold infinity in the palm of your hand / And eternity in an hour," I had been dimly conscious of an unresolvable conundrum at the core of life. But I could not touch it with words, and paid only glancing attention to it as time passed, until I started to study and, more particularly, to teach yoga. At that point, the concept of paradox began to pervade everything, from the physical to the mental, the mundane to the sublime. Even my initials—AW—remind me of alpha (α) and omega (Ω), the eternal beginning and end!

I had begun to notice a curious thing as I engaged in the physical practice. I was forced over time to recognize that, while I thought I was doing yoga, somehow it was doing me. In other words, while I shaped my body to the asanas, I found that the practice was reshaping the body and mind. The author of the work suddenly seemed elusive, a state of affairs brought home to me when I realized that, instead of being skeptical about spiritual matters, I had begun to think in terms of an intelligence pervading all things, something I might now call the soul of the universe. But if we look upon yoga as the use of the accessible (the body, the breath, meditation) to reach into and affect the inaccessible (organs, nerves, brain, and subtle centers), can we be surprised that those organs and systems then provide autonomous feedback that influences our disposition and actions? Experiencing these changes marked the beginning of a perplexing inquiry into the nature of doing and nondoing fundamental to karma yoga, and in more general terms the beginning of my inquiry into paradox.

I first encountered yoga when, in my early twenties, I married a man forty years older than I. He was an eccentric French diplomat, a well-known dance critic in Europe, and something of a dreamer, who had read and admired Sir Aurobindo. Every morning he would turn his bath into a simple, elemental ritual of plain washing and ablution, humming and prayer, which he followed with an abbreviated asana practice. I scorned and resisted his activities; he would gently chide me, assuring me that one day I would understand. This amicable standoff was followed by a few unproductive experiments with yoga classes in Paris and Rome. I remained blind to the poetry of the inward locomotion in the poses and the alternately silent or fiery song of the breath. But feeling that it would help my lover with his scoliosis, I went along, finally succumbing to hatha yoga in Munich in 1983. Perhaps it was my pantheistic love of nature that served as a chink in the armor of my skepticism.

Why the poses penetrated my body and mind in a more compelling way on that occasion, who can say? Physical challenge and the acquisition of skill had always appealed to me; I am still exhilarated by mastering a new difficulty or relinquishing an old habit. But the real seduction and pleasure came from a deep, almost cellular experience of release, as if the body were being broken open at its core.

Those first early courses in Munich were followed by classes in New York, an introduction to meditation, several teacher trainings under the aegis of the Sivananda organization and a broader acquaintance with other schools of yoga, as rivalrous as any group of organized religions. The various schools aired their opinions of each other freely. To the Sivananda organization Iyengar yoga was too athletic, to the hard-core Iyengar community Ashtanga was too athletic, and so full circle to the Sivananda style, which was viewed elsewhere as too uneducated and soft. Some of these prejudices have abated to a degree, but fundamental differences in point of view naturally remain, giving each form its character, virtue and, perhaps, its limitation. These differences mattered to me in part because the experience of contradiction has been a fruitful one. Ashtanga yoga, for example, calls for the almost constant holding of mula bandha (or root lock. T. K. V. Desikachar disagrees with this approach. The Iyengar method calls for shoulderstand to follow headstand without exception, while the reverse order is written into the closing poses of every Ashtanga series, although a closer examination caused me to note that jalandhara bandha, or chin lock, in one of the lotus poses following headstand, provides both a counterpose and the cooling effect of shoulderstand. In fact, as I looked at the first three Ashtanga series, I observed that they all move methodically from the base of the spine in the standing poses to the crown of the head. These differences have challenged me to try to understand the forms I have worked with the most, and to consider the paradox of their irreconcilable viabilities.

I entered into a direct experience of the opposing forces of tradition and change when, after several years of teaching at the Sivananda Center in New York, I had begun to feel the need for both deeper insight into the poses and a more dynamic approach. I was given to understand that studying or teaching elsewhere would undermine the unique quality of the Sivananda teaching, a point of view that I understood and rejected, by resigning, at the same time. At some point, we decide whether to accept a teaching in its entirety or not.

Thanks to an introduction from David Life, I began to study Iyengar yoga with Kevin Gardiner, a passionate teacher with a love and knowledge of detail, indeed of micromovements in the poses. The intelligence, wit, and intensity of his teaching marked a turning point in my education, sustained by subsequent study with Mary Dunn. By discovering new depths of physical precision I was invited to recognize more clearly the unexplored fields of knowledge that lay before me and what I then viewed as the limitations of my own practice. I began a more definite inquiry into the character of the poses, their effects, and their aesthetic content. Just as the study of grammar and rhetoric can enhance one's appreciation of great poetry, so too with the analysis of poses and their alignment.

The body and mind as a unified field, a miraculously subtle network, is no longer a theory for me but a full realization. This understanding, expressed by the extension of the mind deep into every cell of the body through, for example, the nervous and endocrine systems (there is even "brain matter" in the gut), lends weight to the importance of cultivating equanimity. We, or at least I, chronically underestimate the power of the mind to affect ourselves and others. And yet our own brains sculpt themselves into synaptic channels or "valleys," as Guy Claxton calls the grooves of our memory in *Hare Brain, Tortoise Mind.* To the yoga student, these channels are the well-known samskaras of the sutras, deepened and replenished by thoughts and actions, or deprived of their force by channeling mental energy elsewhere.

By the summer of 1998, a desire to learn more about the "hidden" body led me to participate in one of Gil Hedley's noted nonmedical dissection workshops. Down in the bowels of the New Jersey School of Medicine and Dentistry, in a large, cold room, I and twelve fellow students dissected the cadavers of a man and a woman, both of whom who appeared to be in their late sixties or early seventies. According to protocol, we were told nothing about them, which lent a sense of mystery and heightened curiosity to the undertaking, particularly since our indefatigable teacher challenged us to discover the probable cause of death.

I felt enormous tenderness for these two departed beings, provoked first by the fact of their deaths and their gift of themselves to the pursuit of knowledge, and then because of the intimacy of our contact. All their wounds and illnesses were revealed over time: his greenish, cancerous, crumbling cervical rib, the brilliant red and green colors in the subcutaneous tissues indicating chemotherapy, the huge blood clot in his stomach speaking of a last hemorrhage; the mottled pink hemispheres of her brain signaling a stroke, and the resulting badly torn ligaments and cartilage in her knee.

At each level of the dissection we paused in meditation around the corpses. Gil invited us to sympathetically experience the dead bodies and our own at whatever layer we were working on. Can it seem possible to find the flayed body, clothed only in its pinkish, yellowish fat, as adorable, as lovable as a favorite plush toy? And yet I did. When Gil pushed us to explore our feelings about the fat layer in our own body, it left me with a sense of fluidity and softness. But, when we had removed the fat and reached the large muscle groups, I experienced a disturbing

awareness of stored anger and tension in mine.

The neat laying out of muscles, sinews, vessels, and organs in anatomical illustrations in no way conveys the difficulty of trying to sort out the individual elements, whether following one single nerve through half the body or separating one muscle from its almost indistinguishable neighbor. The "fluffing" of the muscles, as this process of separation was called, caused them to hang from their attachments almost like garlands. Since we could freely handle the cadavers, I was able to see the shape of the muscles of the woman's flayed arms and legs when placed in the classical, spiraling position emphasized in Iyengar yoga (and the spiral *is* one of yoga's particular secrets). The muscles ceased to hang and pressed deeply to the bone as they twisted tight like a cloth being wrung out. I thought of Virabhadrasana I, or the first of the warrior poses, and of the surge of energy and strength I have so often experienced while executing the pose, due in part to this essential, spiraling action of the back leg and extended arms. This same extension of the arms markedly affects the lungs as well, as I was about to find out.

Before beginning the dissection, we had looked carefully at the bodies and gently moved the limbs, looking for signs of imbalance or injury. One of the things we noticed was a stiffness in the right shoulder of the woman. In itself this was fairly banal, but by the time we had cut away the ribs and exposed the lungs, we saw something that gave us food for thought: the lung had adhered to the upper chest wall, directly beneath the frozen shoulder. In other words, either the physical immobility had moved inwards, affecting the lung itself or, conversely, a problem in the lung had affected the shoulder. Each step of the dissection seemed to dramatize a significant aspect of the asanas, in this case either the stretching and massaging of the organs through the action of the limbs or the use of the breath to produce free movement. Later, Gil illustrated the influence of one part of the body on another, encouraging us to feel the delicate movement in the sacrum of the male corpse as he pulled hard on the dura surrounding and protecting the brain. It was a disturbingly life-like and revealing sensation, pointing to the deep cerebral action of forward bends, for example. While one scarcely needs such experiences to trust the profound effects of yoga, they make an indelible impression, underscoring the lessons learned through other means.

As we eviscerated the abdomen, attempting to remove entire parts of the digestive system intact (such as the kidneys, ureters, and bladder), I was belatedly moved to think about the place-ment of organs in relation to the vayus, or subtle energies gov-erning the body's functions. To observe that the water element embodied by the kidneys, for example, lay behind the perito-neum (the membrane lining and dividing the abdominal cavity), while fire, embodied in the digestive tract, lay in front of it suddenly rendered more vivid the traditional view that an as-cending solar energy, or prana, governs the front of the body, while apana, or the descending lunar energy dominates the back.

When, in the final moments of our exploration, I held the min-iscule pituitary gland on the tip of my index finger, I was moved to tears—so small, so delicate, so powerful. Gil pointed out its placement directly on the chiasma of the optic nerve, confirming for me the importance of the quality of one's gaze not just during practice, but at all times. The relation of the gaze to one's state of mind, the influence of the aesthetic quality of the thing viewed, the stimulation of the optic nerve through eye exercises—all these are reasons for which I teach "serene gazing" as a first principle of practice. It is a gaze characterized by its distribution from peripheral to central, or both focused and not focused, in a face verging on a smile. This reciprocity between the face and brain cannot be overemphasized. Smiling itself has been shown to help with depression and to have specific effects on, for example, blood flow to the head. As a counterpart to this practice of serene gazing, I look in all the asanas for both Tadasana and Savasana, or life and death, effort and grace.

It was almost inevitable, when we looked for the last time at the remains of our friends, that we dwell on mortality and immortality, the nature of human identity and its location (or absence of precise location), and many other things both nameable and confusedly wordless. As the bodies disappeared, their human individuality steadily blossomed. It was not unlike cutting back a plant only to find that, without the leaves, the essence of "plant" nonetheless survives. At what point did the individual cease, or not cease? This was perhaps the closest one could come to the practical and exclusively physical application of Neti Neti in jnana yoga, the exercise of "I am neither this, nor that," engaged in with the hope of discovering one's changeless identity. The only difference was that we were quite literally applying this methodical elimination of every mutable, transient part of the body to two corpses.

Through this intellectual inquiry of jnana yoga, or the "yoga of wisdom," into the nature of one's identity by an elimination of all that is transient or changeable, from the cells of the body to one's opinion about the existence of Santa Claus, I have apprehended if not realized an imperishable state beyond the limitations of whatever I perceive to be my personal identity. The physical practice, too, has afforded moments of illumination about the power of the poses to reveal the heart to the so-called rational mind. In relation to what, for example, am I experiencing such gratitude and calm in child's pose? What ineffable presence fills the emptied mind? Savasana provides the final lesson. I now teach an annual "practice of death" on Good Friday, an ecumenical invitation to experience through the body and the breath the approach of death. Investigating and accepting the inevitable loss of the body through corpse pose turns out to be a deeply reassuring practice. Insofar as it provokes this kind of inquiry into the nature of the permanent and impermanent, jnana yoga is also a practice of death, as in fact are all traditions in which one is invited to shed the limitations of one's identity.

I look upon the answers I have reached at this point, and even some of the questions, as working hypotheses only. As my practice of yoga has deepened, to those questions have come both increasingly temporary and contradictory answers, tempered by an occasional and restful plateau of certainty. Just as the alpinist's view changes with each stage of the ascent, so my view has changed with each inbound step.

Yoga has shown me in a visceral way that there are powerful fields of mental energy fueled by the tensions of viable yet seemingly irreconcilable opposites—or paradox. They are one of the hidden sources of life's flowering, as important as sunlight and water. While I may still flee ambiguity and difficulty in my life, I have nonetheless come to understand that a willingness to embrace ambiguity, to cultivate paradox, is essential to my practice and spiritual growth.

As a result, I have tried to form some idea of what paradox is to our brain. An analogy came to me from my former discipline as an art historian, and particularly as a historian of sculpture. A famous debate comparing the virtues of painting and sculpture took on dramatic proportions during the Renaissance. Leonardo and Michelangelo figured prominently in it. Among the chief points in favor of painting was that the subject could be assimilated at once, whereas time and displacement were required for appreciating sculpture. The same may be said of different "thought forms." Logic, while still taking time to process, is a linear, sequential, or two-dimensional problem for what I call the three-dimensional mind, as opposed to the elusive paradox, grasped by the mind like a three-dimensional object, one side at a time. With that in mind, I might consider free will and destiny a continuum called "choice" with different authors. At one extreme lies the individual and at the other something like the organizing principle of the universe. Paradox is like a three-dimensional thought form in relation to a three-dimensional perceptual system. Only in the fourth dimension, or the supramental state, can the difficulty be resolved. From this arises the use of paradox-like Zen koans (e.g., A girl is crossing the road. Is she the older or younger sister?) to precipitate the stultified brain into a new realm of understanding.

I quickly grasped that one could not hope to solve a paradox in the immediate moment by focused intellectual examination. The more I tried to define the parameters, the more the center evaporated, and vice versa. A more peripheral mental gaze, to use the analogy of sight again, tends to reduce the mental friction of coping with paradox, while leaving room for insight. In other words, I can invite paradox to do its work by entertaining it in the mind as often as possible in a simultaneously focused and unfocused way (developing the equivalent of a paradoxical state to begin the approach to paradox), feeling its discomfiting presence until it works its magic and yields a more subtle instrument.

Thousands of years ago, the Bhagavad Gita addressed the matter indirectly. Presenting the most prominent vehicles of self-inquiry and realization, among them karma yoga or the yoga of self-less, self-full action, the Gita shows Krishna guiding Arjuna into the same thorny thicket of paradox we find ourselves in here, but with some invaluable markers and goals, the ultimate one being transparency to the divine. The concept of practice in itself seems arduous, whereas non-doership may be viewed as a state of emptiness, or transparency at the heart of action. At this point one might even consider the notion of a practice irrelevant, something burdened by puritanical obligation, or yet another obstruction to and deferring of the ever-present truth which cannot be achieved effortfully. Whichever way one turns the word *practice* around, some form of impetus or desire is at the root of our efforts or nonefforts. And still, as has so often been said, only the ground may be prepared, giving rise to the delicate play of effort and grace.

balancing acts: two views on ashtanga

Janet Bowdan and Roz Peters

I am not fluent in Sanskrit

My teacher advises the new Ashtanga students, "Instead of jumping to chattaranga, lower yourself like this: knees, chest, chin." She says sympathetically, "When you get tired, rest in downward dog." She says, "After practice, take a long hot bath. Be good to yourself." I really like my teacher, but I don't remember her taking this gentle approach with those of us who started in her first class here three years ago. I remember her being especially gleeful as she called out, "Navasana!" and watched us struggle to maintain our balance. I know she didn't use that "knees, chest, chin" thing until a good nine months afterward, after we'd already developed enough upper-body strength not to need to think, "We can't stay here! What do you mean, another sun salutation A? We still have to do all five Bs!" It wasn't so much physical pain (though it hurt, building muscle) as a conflict of the mind against the body: What am I doing here? Why am I staying in this position?

Doing Ashtanga makes me happy, and I'm still wondering how, when it's so much work. Should I do more yoga to be even happier? Now my teacher suggests, "The teacher-training course starts next weekend."

"I don't want to teach," I say. What I mean is, I don't want to teach yoga. I already teach four English courses a semester.

"You don't have to teach," she says. "It deepens your regular practice!"

Cost aside ($1,750 is not trivial, even if, like one of my friends in Boston, I could offer enough "kick-ass yoga" classes to replenish my bank account in no time flat), two hundred hours of weekends aside (When would I correct papers? Do laundry? See my boyfriend?), I have to struggle just to maintain a regular practice. "Remember to breathe" is my current mantra.

My cousin Roz, on the other hand, teaches yoga for a living, and I can see how it is possible to become so enamored of yoga that it would become a way of life.

Roz and I have been writing each other across the Atlantic since we were eleven. We wrote long letters about family, school, and what we thought we might want to do with our lives, which kept changing. We sent postcards from places we each wished the other could have seen. It occurred to me when Roz's postcards started to come from Greece and India that yoga might be a rather nice thing to do, if it gave me an excuse to travel to these schools. Yoga as a topic had crept in quite gradually; it took me some time to realize Roz was talking about it as the center of her life because she kept referring to it as her "practice," which I associated with playing the piano.

Practice is basically the correct effort required to move toward, reach, and maintain the state of yoga.

—T. K. V. Desikachar, *The Heart of Yoga*

To: Janet Bowdan	Date: Friday, 16 June 2000
From: Roz Peters	Subject: Yoga 2

Dear Janet,

Ignore previous e-mail, written while waiting for printer to disgorge your first piece. As my perceptions change almost daily, here are yesterday's quick quick, before the next sea change. You were asking what ambitions we had when we started doing yoga? "Started" is the key here—to rest, relax, at a stressful point in my life; grand ambition came later (find God) via vanity (o wow, look at my biceps) and a way of life (who needs a career when there's India and travel, o joy, irresponsibility, freedom at last)—15 years on, I'd say the aspiration (coward's version of goal?) is to be happy, to find balance in my life [samtosha], to avoid striving. And the gain is the moment I feel content (and it may not last all day), but o it's wonderful when it happens.

To: Roz Peters	Date: June 16, 2000
From: Janet Bowdan	Subject: Re: Yoga 2

My ambition was to gain time somehow, make that moment of content spill into the rest of my life. I felt I was losing years, and you told me that Pattabhi Jois would occasionally change the clocks forward or back just by a few minutes to teach his Western students about impatience. When they came to class (4:30 A.M.?), he'd ask them, "Why so early?" or, "Why so late?" You said, and it helped:

To: Janet Bowdan	Date: 17 June 2000
From: Roz Peters	Subject: Time is

East is geared toward awareness of infinity, which is reflected in the pace of daily life and used to justify the hiccups and irregularities which might infuriate an impatient Western "every second counts" believer. It does count, but in context: It's one second in bazillions since the Universe began. . . .

If you can't resolve a problem/achieve a goal in this life, so you work towards it, and perhaps be reincarnated in a better state to achieve it next time. During each cycle of each planet, there are appropriate/auspicious times for all things, depending on your horoscope, the seasons, and countless other variables. During each day the sun's strength dictates appropriate times for different occupations: the hours around sunrise and sunset are most auspicious for yoga, around sunset more so for meditation; the full heat of the day is inappropriate for food, sleep, or sex. Consult your personal Vedic astrologer for advice on when to do anything!

Yoga first took hold of me in 1992, a first taste of that contentment—not achievement, just acceptance of how life was. I have a ceaselessly moving mind, housed in a sluggish old body. Yoga drew me in with offers of even a moment's waking reprieve for that mind, and a few knock-on benefits of improved energy levels, posture, et al. It worked. I'm still doing it. It's a hurdle to get the body to join in some days. But if it won't, the mind won't get there, either. The sloth in me looked for simpler, easier routes—and yes, a decent bottle of wine may bring merriment, but hasn't quite the same benefits. Onward with the yoga. Life is hard. Reread last line until you truly accept it. Accept that and everything else gets easier.

To: Roz Peters   Date: June 18, 2000
From: Janet Bowdan   Subject: Starting yoga

I started yoga in 1993, when I was teaching in Louisiana. I had friends, but I was lonely anyway. I also had tendinitis from correcting five or six composition classes' worth of papers each semester. You'd been writing me about yoga—you'd found something in it, a solid form of hope, maybe, which I needed, and a woman I knew was offering to teach it. I don't know what kind it was; she'd studied in some ashram in Venezuela. So I started. The class was in a peaceful, sunny room with huge windows. Rabbits hopped around outside. I'd never, ever been good at anything requiring athletic talent; I don't have a brain and body that mesh intuitively. My brain may grasp an idea, but repeating a sequence and reminding myself "outward rotation" or "exhale" is the only way my body will learn to follow that idea. But I had some flexibility, and that was enough for me to be amazed at my progress, to feel happier about myself. That kept me looking for yoga teachers when I moved to Massachusetts. By then you were doing Ashtanga; mostly what I found were New Agey courses—relaxing, but no focus. Then an Ash-tanga class began here, and I found it instantly engaging. I could feel myself getting stronger. I was impressed with my teacher's strength and stam-ina; I thought I could work on this sequence until I got it right, 20 or 30 years from now, perhaps. Now I'm a bit worried that I won't have the patience to keep up, won't be satisfied with the promises of yoga before I have some return for my work.

To: Janet Bowdan   Date: 18 June 2000
From: Roz Peters   Subject: Yoga 4?

What promises? My teacher always said, "Do your practice and all is coming." At first I thought, great, I keep on doing these asanas and I reach perfect happiness, the end of the rainbow. Some years later, it occurs to me that I may have been overoptimistic in my definition of "all"—all hell breaks loose, all things good and bad come to pass—but just possibly, I'm better equipped to deal with it "all," now.

A more literal answer—yoga's "returns" or siddhis—literally, "perfec-tions"—include enhanced pranic and psychic capacity, paranormal and supernormal accomplishments, complete control over mind and prana (seeing through walls and into the future, understanding birdsong, being in two places at once, overcoming death). While I may have my moments, I'm not there yet and I don't expect to be—yoga is a lifetime's work.

To: Roz Peters   Date: June 18, 2000
From: Janet Bowdan   Subject: Yes but

Yes, but you have to do it all the time. There must be some hope that makes (Ashtanga) yoga practitioners redesign their lives to incorporate a regular practice (two hours daily).

To: Janet Bowdan   Date: 19 June 2000
From: Roz Peters   Subject: Yoga 3 or 4

Dear correspondent, I can read your mind, because I've been there. They're very driven, like any learning curve, in the early days; the speed at which their practice grows and changes is great. I was that person once; later, realising I'm here for the long haul, I'm grateful to be motivated to get on my mat at all, not for a period of fixed length, or for a practice of fixed name. Just grateful. Why? Those elusive rewards, that contentment.

| To: Roz Peters | Date: June 20, 2000 |
| From: Janet Bowdan | Subject: Yoga question |

I wondered, being somewhat tempted myself, what lures some yoga students to become teachers (or to intensify their practice by taking extra classes, going on yoga retreats, taking teacher-training courses). What I saw of your decision was that, after a long internal debate on what to do, you planned to teach secondary education; you'd had the whole certification program organized before you went off to a last holiday in Mysore. When you came back, you scrapped the whole scheme and announced you were going to teach yoga. The essential core of that idea may get complicated—corrupted, even—by questions of insurance, pension plans, assessment. . . . But obviously you want to teach what you love, to spend your time learning more about it and to share it.

Yoga . . . is a practical method for making one's life purposeful, useful and noble.

—B. K. S. Iyengar, *Light on the Yoga Sutras of Patanjali*

Roz's letters showed me how much work it was to set up a career teaching yoga, how hard to achieve balance between earning a living and living a fulfilling life.

1997: Roz on Yoga

20 January 1997

Dear Janet,

(written on the back of two pages from *The Complete Illustrated Book of Yoga* by Vishnudevananda, illustrating Paschimottanasana)

I've been writing endless yoga essays—cutting out and gluing up graphic illustrations of hairy man bending forwards (see over), etc. The course is good fun, and I'm learning more about anatomy and physiology than I ever did at school. A lot of people have made New Year's resolutions to go to yoga: My classes are much fuller. And I'm in discussion with (is that the correct Hollywood term?) three more venues regarding setting up more classes—all N. London, v. handy. . . .

Enjoy the new term and if you are back at yoga classes, I trust the teacher entertains you.

STOP PRESS: India May–Aug only: a record short stay. How disciplined I am becoming.

13 March 1997
Dear Janet,

(written on the back of publicity photos and a flyer for a Level II Ashtanga vinyasa yoga course with Roz Peters: "Roz is a member of the European Union of Ashtanga Vinyasa Yoga and is studying for the British Wheel of Yoga Diploma.")

Here I am, sitting at my desk, trying to take my mind off tomorrow (unusually), but I'm having my teaching assessed for a diploma I'm taking, and the prospect makes me nervous. I've been busy with classes lately, and my latest time-consumer is using Mira's PC to prepare timetables and adverts, etc. See over if bored.

My own classes go well. . . . I have a new venture forthcoming with a very expensive health club. On my way to discuss terms, my exhaust fell off on the motorway: I must have been the most uncalm, late, and anxious yoga teacher they'd ever met when I arrived. But I'm going to be lecturing on "yoga and health" and give individual tutorials.

I'm indeed heading for Mysore. My circumstances and motivation have altered considerably since my last trip. Now it's a HOLIDAY, from teaching, from keeping house, to see my teacher, to do my own practice and recharge my batteries. . . . The prospect of heat, monsoon, Indian food, and time to read is just marvelous.

I'm delighted that your teaching continues rewarding. I wish for your sake grading and preparation weren't so time-consuming though. I know I'm happier on a lower income and fewer core work hours, but that's my choice.

23 April 1997
Dear Janet,

I took a stupid risk and popped my knee. I'm still hopping a bit, much less painful now, and am off for three weeks of leisure and no yoga to Mysore.

8 May 1997, Mysore
Dear Janet,

I'm so happy to be here and appreciative of my surroundings.

I reckoned that in eighteen months of continuous teaching, I'd only had two weeks of vacation [in addition to Xmas and Easter]. No wonder I was shattered.

I went to see my dear old teacher here: H's recently celebrated sixty years in the classroom: no retirement in sight. We had such a valuable conversation: I was concerned about a) my lousy knee and b) my lousy teaching thanks to the lousy knee. He put my mind at rest on both scores. I walked away understanding what Catholics see in absolution.

And so I'm back on my yoga mat. I'm only here for three weeks, but the journey was worthwhile for that conversation alone.

Essentially, the teacher's recommendations were carry on doing and teaching yoga, but take it slow.

My room (with all-marble bathroom, and view of coconut palms through the monkey bars) costs £2.30/night.

27 November 1997
Dear Janet,

I seem to spend a day each week on a computer at the moment. I've written nine of twenty essays for the yoga diploma course I'm on, which continues its attempts to rule my life (just say NO).

So, I've been enjoying life and spending (almost) as much as I earn lately. How will I have enough for my next Mysore sortie at this rate, and who will live here? Await next gripping installment.

Dharanasu ca yogyata manasah: **The mind also becomes fit for concentration.**
—Yoga Sutras of Patanjali (II.53)

1998: Janet on Yoga

January 1998
Dear Roz,

I've been doing yoga in class but not out (no discipline, no sticky mat).

March 1998

Dear Roz,

We're on spring break! I corrected papers, met my mother for lunch and then vacuumed before going back to Amherst for yoga.

Three of my colleagues went to England over break, two to Paris, two to South America. You're in India. Right now, home is exotic enough for me.

June 1998

Dear Roz,

I have been doing yoga about twice a week, an Ashtanga class on Saturdays and an Iyengar class either on Tuesday night or Thursday morning, whichever I end up managing to get to (a matter of exhaustion rather than schedule).

November 1998

Dear Roz,

I've been thinking of writing you for more than a month, but I haven't had spare time. Well, I can see your expression now. But really, it's not that bad. It's much better than this summer, when I had enough time to be aware of how crunched I'd be this year. Now I'm in the thick of it, I'm feeling more productive. I've been fitting some fun in, too. The reason I didn't write you in October was that I took two weekend yoga workshops, one very relaxing with Judith Lasater—many restorative poses and some Zen stories.

The next yoga weekend was an introductory Ashtanga workshop with my regular teacher, Patty. For me it was a long, slowed-down version of class (five hours Saturday, five hours Sunday), with some background. My father took it, too, and he really enjoyed it. In fact, he muttered for several weeks about fitting Ashtanga into his routine—problem is, it cuts into his karate time. The Wednesday night class will start in January: The teacher takes the Saturday class once a month now, and he pays attention to detail, very enthusiastic about any improvement. Patty is good, somewhat more severe; her Saturday class is serious. I suspect she's more cheerful in her Monday class, a slower, gentler approach to Ashtanga. The Wednesday class should be a happy medium.

The local public radio station (meaning, classical music) asked me to talk on air to persuade people to pledge, so I did. I told a yoga story: The day before, I said, I'd been at my yoga class (the other reason I come into Amherst at eight on a weekend morning), and at one point I realized that I was standing on one leg trying to get my other leg up to touch my nose, and twenty other people were doing the same thing, and I realized that people will do a lot when something is important to them. (At this point the two radio professionals talking with me knew where I was headed.) And you feel the benefits of yoga almost instantly, I said: you have more energy, you feel better about yourself, you feel you know more . . . very like the benefits from pledging to public radio. And some of the things you do that are impor-

tant are hard, like trying to get your leg up to your nose, or—one of my favorites—getting your leg behind your ear—and some are easy, like calling the station and charging a pledge.

A woman who goes to my Saturday yoga class heard that and was delighted. I didn't ask her if she'd pledged.

Only connect.

—E. M. Forster, *Howards End*

To: Roz Peters   Date: July 10, 2000
From: Janet Bowdan   Subject: The business of yoga

I suspect it changes the practice of and perspective on yoga to be a professional rather than an amateur. Does it?

To: Janet Bowdan   Date: 11 July 2000
From: Roz Peters   Subject: Water gardens

My practice hasn't changed *because* I teach now—it changes because life changes and because it is a reflection and part of life. Yoga teaches me to observe, balance, connect. On a practical note, there were times when I was first trying to make a living teaching, and taught so many hours that there weren't quite enough (enthusiastic, motivated) hours left to get on my own mat. That was just sad, and made the whole exercise feel futile. Took a good while to get a balance back.

To: Roz Peters   Date: July 12, 2000
From: Janet Bowdan   Subject: In balance

I believe it's precisely in not thinking about yoga as something to teach that I approach "balance": For you it seems yoga has become the world, absorbing everything (you see everything from its light). For me, teaching is already a rubric split and in contention with poetry: What I experience I immediately think of turning to use—how can I write about this? (Also, when can I find time to write?)

To: Janet Bowdan From: Roz Peters
Date: 14 July 2000 Subject: Reverence for the world

Our different worldviews, and healthily different. For you, everything is potential poetic inspiration. For me, I'm sure there was a time when there was a) yoga and b) rest of life, but having spent more time looking at the philosophical dimensions of yoga, feeling that I agree with its logic, it becomes excessively hard work to try to keep an increasingly artificial divide.

To: Roz Peters Date: July 15, 2000
From: Janet Bowdan Subject: Problem

Does the teacher need to lead a lifestyle wholly consistent with yogic philosophies in order to be a good teacher, in order for the student to be fulfilled?

To: Janet Bowdan Date: 16 July 2000
From: Roz Peters Subject: Honesty

The eternal dilemma: Do I practice what I preach? For me, honesty is crucial, though students may be taken aback occasionally—"Do you do that every day?" one will gasp, amazed, at a first lesson. "No'," I'll reply. I make sure to distinguish between what's ideal according to yogic tradition, and balancing that with living in a Western world, not an ashram. I don't aspire to wake at four A.M. so as to be in tune with nature at the most sacred hour of the day, though I'm sure it would feel extraordinary if I did, nor to eat before sundown (it gets dark in London by four P.M. in winter—who am I trying to kid here?).

I tried getting up 4 A.M., practice 4.30–7, office by 8.45, home at 7 P.M. bed at 9 P.M. It was a strictly temporary arrangement: six months max. I salute anyone who can maintain that practice for a lifetime—though it taught me things and steered me to make choices.

I teach three evenings a week, every week. Traditionally one wouldn't practice on a full or new moon—but the classes are there on the calendar—I make students aware of traditions and the logic behind them, and let them make up their own minds. As for a student's fulfillment, a teacher leads the way—but that's up to them.

So dear reader, advice unasked for, I know: Set yourself achievable goals. Five minutes of yoga for the next few days, ten and twenty will follow in their own time. Better than two hours on Monday, stiff on Tuesday, can't face it on Wednesday, consolation beer Thursday, forget about it the rest of the week, and try again Monday.

Yoga comes in many forms, soft, meditative, dynamic, prayer, sheer hard work—each to his own. My yoga mat works for me, for now. Not necessarily always and not necessarily for you. Seek and you shall find. Enjoy.

To: Roz Peters   Date: July 18, 2000
From: Janet Bowdan   Subject: & happy

Well, my yoga mat seems to work best for me when it's facing other mats (and yogis). I need yoga to be social. Maybe this is a good type of peer pressure, like a hand keeping you balanced.

Something bothers me: I keep hearing you say that you don't see yourself as so far advanced or privileged over your students and yet you have a guru voice often that corrects what I say or suggests what was obvious or goes into a lecture.

To: Janet Bowdan   Date: 19 July 2000
From: Roz Peters   Subject: Changes

Oh sorry, Janet, brevity of response vs. true face-to-face dialogue (with accompanying facial expressions—I suspect I'm equally dogmatic in class, it just comes over better . . . .). Isn't it possible to be confident about what we know, and equally sure that there's an awful lot we don't? I still agree with myself from an Ashtanga perspective: If I'm asked questions about Ashtanga, I endeavour to pass on information as accurately as I can, in the same way it was given to me. Hence the dogmatic attitude. Although I'm perfectly happy to play with other styles of yoga (which inevitably and perfectly acceptably mix postures from all sorts of Ashtanga series into one practice). Don't go looking to me for logic!

Yoga, like life, is a long, winding, far from linear path, and no two people are ever going to be at exactly the same point on it at the same time. Reading everything you write, it's like conversing with myself at a different point on the same path: I can only tell you what I feel—I have no expectation that you'll instantly switch motorway lanes and be at the same point as me—why should you, especially if your point on the road is one where you're happy and mine has no advantage whatever over yours. Nor, however, can I undo the experiences I've had and line my viewpoint up with yours. It is entirely plausible for both our standpoints to exist at the same time and both to make sense.

To: Roz Peters   Date: July 20, 2000
From: Janet Bowdan   Subject: Hi

I find myself in the yoga class having some revelation and being distracted by wanting to write to you about it, or to use it in a poem. But I've always found distractions, above my head if not in what I have to do, once I leave class. (All the ceilings of my yoga classrooms have been fascinating, especially the one surrounded by little gilt lions' heads, each holding a light bulb in its mouth.)

Besides distraction, there is fear to overcome. It took me three years to do a handstand. Was that mostly a matter of convincing myself I could? I can now reach around my back and grasp my left toe with my right hand; occasionally I can do this on the other side, too. I'm really pleased with these accomplishments, though, and happy I took the time to get there. It's not easy being patient with myself.

My life is much richer outside of class than it was. That might not have happened without yoga, if I hadn't had energy and courage from Ashtanga to change my habits. Class is rich, too: when the breath is right, when we're doing sun salutations together, I feel the way I do when I'm singing, in the middle of a concert with all those voices, all the orchestral instruments, combining to create a whole, lifting me in this music.

So I have to keep going with it, but I don't want to be obsessive; that means not letting Saturday yoga stop me from taking a weekend away now and then. This balance may be something I can only achieve for a few breaths, like a handstand.

Anyone **can practise yoga.**

—Yehudi Menuhin

To: Janet Bowdan | Date: 25 August 2000
From: Roz Peters | Subject: My advice

Yoga has certainly taken over a lot of lives. My advice: Don't let it! Keep a balance with real-world activity; that's the biggest challenge of all.

To: Roz Peters | Date: December 12, 2000
From: Janet Bowdan | Subject: Entertainment

I want to make yoga a part of my real life, not the main point of it. When I actually made it to England and took your class, it was wonderful not just because it produced much laughter and also a brief serenity but also because before it, we had to cope with horrendous London traffic and after it, we feasted on Indian food. Maybe it is the contrast that makes it work for me, like the time we practiced in the garden: lovely, except for the slugs. Remember? After my father saw us, I expected him to get a camera; instead he brought out his dinner and a chair to sit watching us. He was gradually joined by our entire family, so that we became their dinner entertainment. When we finished, they cheered. Every time I do yoga, I feel it's special — I've earned a little applause. We all have.

an insomniac awakes

Lois Nesbitt

Where did it all begin?

Or, more to the point, when did it all begin to fall apart?

Some life changes are easy to trace. We get hit with the unexpected or unplanned—we fall in love, lose a job, suffer an accident—and suddenly drop into a new role, a new identity, a new life. Other changes we plan, choosing to get pregnant, move to a new town, set up a business.

This was different. There I was, thirty-something, living the life of a latter-day New York intellectual, having carefully and painstakingly positioned myself to play this role. I did not realize that I was unhappy; I felt no gnawing emptiness in my gut. I had no sense that my experience was not complete, that I was not "whole."

This may be because above all I was *busy*. I was writing criticism for a slew of art and design magazines, creating and executing conceptual art projects in Europe and the States, editing books and articles, doing studio visits, and giving lectures. Stacks of papers and drawings representing various projects lay arrayed like parquet squares across the floor of my studio apartment, which functioned more as a library/office than a home; books lined the walls. I spent my days writing, creating art, and seeing to the logistics of getting ideas out into the world; my evenings passed in a blur of gallery openings and book parties.

Everybody I knew was doing the same sort of thing, for I had surrounded myself with people whose thoughts and actions coincided with mine.

Still, things began to crumble—or *I* did. The creeping malaise, the piercing melancholy that I had suppressed under a crust of chronic anxiety and activity erupted in insomnia, unidentifiable yet debilitating illnesses, bouts of depression. I found myself in the New York club scene, prowling the night fueled by intoxicants and an unappeasable angst. All was not well in Mudville. My glorious ship was sinking, and I had lost sight of the shore.

Late in the spring of my thirty-third year, Easter weekend to be exact, I awoke Sunday morning distressed over my physical condition. Eating compulsively in a desperate attempt to buoy my flagging energy and drinking at night to sedate the internal demons, I was putting on weight while suffering from malnutrition. My depleted immune system had been fighting the flu for three months, and I spent most days in bed while the projects framing my futon lay untouched.

Back then I awoke most mornings in a state of distress. My first thought was typically, "Oh no . . ." Getting through the day seemed to require heroic effort. But that Easter morning something different happened: a voice inside my head, calm yet stern (and decidedly male), announced:

You're going to have to change.

No specifics, no directives, just one sweeping pronouncement.

Having no spiritual consciousness up to that point, and being more upset about my expanding body than my shrinking spirit, I assumed that the voice was addressing my misguided attempts to nourish myself with poor food and calm myself with alcohol. I knew that the voice had come from *outside* me, or that something from outside had colonized my brain, and for the first time in my self-propelled life, I went outside for help.

I landed in several twelve-step programs, where I learned that the new voice signaled my "spiritual awakening," and that the abysmal decline leading to that morning reverie traced the path to my "spiritual bottom."

I don't know why this information took. My parents are black sheep in conventionally religious families, my mother a lapsed Catholic and my father the atheist/agnostic son of a Presbyterian missionary. I had no religious upbringing, no interest in spiritual inquiry, and a firm belief that when things got scary my mind would save me. But something shifted that Easter morning, and try as I might in the months that followed, there was no going back. Life as I knew it was over. I had landed on alien territory, or, more precisely, the ground had dropped away beneath me and I was in free fall.

Massive parts of my old routine ground to a halt. For the first time in my life, I suffered writer's block. (This essay is the first public document I have produced in the seven years since.) Making art filled me with such anxiety that I stopped soliciting new commissions and fumbled gracelessly through my remaining commitments. Even the editing work, the dullest of my "B jobs," proved taxing, and I watched helpless as deadlines came and went.

Not one to sit still, I reacted with whatever concrete actions I could muster. I filled my days with twelve-step meetings, with calls to my "sponsor," with therapy. "Filled" is not quite accurate: I was lucky if I got to one meeting a day, to therapy twice a week. Mostly I did nothing. Right in the middle of my most productive years, I had been struck still, paralyzed by some invisible stun gun aimed at my heart.

And then one Thursday afternoon I landed in a yoga class, and as clearly as one door had shut, another opened.

> Mr. Duffy lived most of his life a short distance from his body.
> —James Joyce, *Ulysses*

Until that day, I had no real connection to my body. Although I ran, swam, or worked out in spurts, it was more from a sense of duty, another "should" on the laundry list of shoulds that filled my days. I should exercise or my body would get fat, stiff, prematurely old. I should exercise because it quelled the constant anxiety. I should exercise because other people did. (Given my fragile sense of self, doing what other people did provided at least a semblance of security.) For long stretches of time I sat in libraries all day, reading and writing, my only exercise being to haul books back and forth from home.

But about a year before the breakdown (breakthrough?) I started scouting around for a yoga teacher. I had been introduced to yoga as a teenager, while studying art in Provence. The school had hired a teacher from New York to give lessons twice a day. (This was 1976: The art history class produced a "happening" instead of term papers, and yoga was a hip way of getting aspiring young artists to exercise.) Every morning and evening a few of us gathered on the stone terraces overlooking the cherry orchards and vineyards. (The rest declined, preferring late-night bacchanals fueled by the local *gros rouge* and Rolling Stones tapes.) Amid this landscape made famous by Cezanne and Van Gogh, we inhaled and exhaled our way through sun salutations, standing postures, backbends, and inversions.

I was hooked. Ever since childhood I had been escaping my two demons—fear and boredom—by retreating into worlds of my own creating, as I drew or wrote stories or got lost in stories written by others. I had come to France that summer, at the age of sixteen and with my life stretching out before me, to decide whether

I would become an artist. The criteria: Could art absorb me? Could the daily practice of putting brush or graphite or charcoal to paper fend off the discontent that seemed to rise with me every morning and huddle next to me during the night?

That summer art failed me. Too often as I painted or etched or drew I found myself distracted by the familiar internal tyrants: relentless self-criticism, nameless longing, profound dis-ease, a boredom so pernicious I just wanted the day to end, and then the next, and the next, until my life itself ended.

But the hours of yoga were different. While I bent and stretched and balanced and breathed the voices got a little softer, time hung a little less heavy. I was here, in my physical body, and not wanting out. This was new.

> *Yogas citta vrtti nirodhah.*
> (The restraint of the modifications of the mind-stuff is yoga.)
> —Patanjali, Yoga Sutras (I.2)

Summer ended, and I went home. For the next few months I diligently practiced what I had learned of yoga on my parents' living room rug. But just as I tried in vain to transport the tangible ingredients of that golden summer back into the mid-Atlantic fall, nibbling tasteless croissants packed in plastic from the local Giant Food, I found that yoga suffered in transit.

The demands of my American high school life began to intrude on my yoga. No one near me in those days thought that yoga was anything more than an exotic pastime I'd picked up overseas. Certainly no one suggested that yoga could be a "full-time" thing, a lifestyle, even (as it is for many today) a career path. Having eliminated "artist" from my future, I threw myself into academics. Getting into a good college consumed me. Yoga, and with it that sweet taste of serenity, went by the wayside.

> I think, therefore I am.
> —René Descartes, *Discourse on Method*

Without the fine thread of hatha yoga to anchor me to my body, I slipped more deeply into the life of the mind. Descartes's disembodied thinker struck me as an apt definition of human exis-

tence (later I developed a strong affinity for the paraplegic rant-
ers of Beckett's plays and novels): As far as I was concerned, the
real "action" happened in the brain. Consciousness as I knew it
carried on independent of the body, what Yeats somewhere referred to as "the dying animal." I reflexively accepted the Western philosophic predilection for separating mind and body and
for seeing mind as clearly the superior of the two. I created a lifestyle that supported this view: by the time I got to graduate
school at Princeton, I had honed my daily routine to ten hours in
the library, broken up by occasional meals at the student center
across the quad. I had little time for other people, and no patience
with the body's seemingly incessant demands for food, for clean
clothes, for sex, for sleep. When I arrived at the library each day I
would slump down in an oversized armchair, a hassock under
my feet. With my body draped over the upholstery like a throw
rug, my mind was free to wander.

And wander I did. For seven years I read, studied languages,
wrote, lectured, taught. I dabbled in art history, architecture,
philosophy, linguistics, literary theory, modern and ancient languages and literatures. Unwilling to commit to a single academic department, I finally enrolled in the comparative literature program, which allowed me to cross disciplines, languages,
and periods as long as I could rationalize the connections.

It was a heady time. I got so absorbed in the books I was reading that fictional characters began to replace real people in my
dreams (Odysseus made epic appearances). I even dreamed in
foreign languages, depending on what I was studying any given
day. My ties to daily life in that colonial New Jersey town grew
more and more tenuous; my ties to *myself* began to strain.

Paradoxically, the more I lost myself in the writings of others,
the more I fixated on the notion of autobiography. I had allowed
my life to grow smaller and smaller, leaving me less and less to
tell, yet I felt compelled to get it down on paper, to identify myself.

Yet this "self" proved elusive. I was instinctively attracted to
modern writers who questioned linear narrative form and, by
implication, the coherent hero, the continuous "self" or person-

ality that gathers wisdom as it moves through a series of life experiences. I wrote:

> Life is not like that; my life is not like that. Rather, it is something much more complicated, series of recurrences, redundancies, hapless repetitions, absolute shocks and surprises, long spells of nothingness, overlays and overlaps the intricacies of which defy any graphic representation. Everything that has happened to me is "with" me now, in me, part of me, yet nothing could be more true of life than that it is one prolonged attrition, one unbroken series of losses in which everything we once had is sucked off into some irretrievable oblivion, and it is only through contrasting situations or uncanny repetitions that we remember anything that has come before (from my *Autobiography: Fiction*, 1989).

I gravitated toward literary sketches of this unstable self. *Vie de Henry Brulard* (Life of Henry Brulard) ostensibly presents an autobiography, yet in fact this text about the life of "Henry Brulard" was penned by a man named Henri Beyle writing under the pseudonym of Stendhal. All three names appear in the text, creating a tangled web of identities fictional and "real." Moreover, none of the three maintains a fixed identity; each evolves over the course of the text like the changing patterns of a kaleidoscope. *"Mais quel est ce caractère? Je serais bien en peine de le dire* (But what is this character? I would be at great pains to say)," laments the author. He senses that he will never, through writing, penetrate to the core of his being. Perhaps that core does not exist.

> Digressions, incontestably, are the sunshine,—they are the life, the soul of reading;—take them out of this book, for instance, you might as well take the book along with them.
>
> —Laurence Sterne, *The Life and Opinions of Tristram Shandy*

English novelist Laurence Sterne, writing some years earlier, lampooned the whole notion of penning one's life in another faux autobiography, *The Life and Opinions of Tristram Shandy*. In fact, in the course of this windy two-volume work, the narrator never advances beyond the physical circumstances of his own birth. This struck me as hilarious, but it also struck a chord. I discovered about this time why I had always had trouble reading: I couldn't stick with *any* linear narrative. I subjected each assertion a writer made to an exhaustive internal debate, which then led me to pursue various tangents that carried me far from the instigating text. To paraphrase another modern writer, the center would not hold.

Character seems to drain out of many literary protagonists in the modern period, propelling early-twentieth-century novelist Robert Musil to title one of his novels *A Man without Qualities.* The chain of fiction's characterless characters culminates in Samuel Beckett's trilogy *Molloy, Malone Dies, The Unnamable,* which traces the dissolution of any coherent narrator. The Unnamable can't muster even the illusion of coherence: "It has not yet been our good fortune to establish with any degree of accuracy what I am, where I am, whether I am words among words, or silence in the midst of silence, to recall only two of the hypotheses launched in this connection."

This radical collapse of certainty, this spiral into infinite questioning, represents more than the breakdown of "whole" characters in fiction. It signals an ontological/epistemological crisis. Who are we? Where did we come from? How can we ever know? Ask away, in a godless modern world, as these authors do—no reassuring answers emerge. And this inability to define the self, to know the self, broadens to the more profound inability to "know" anything. This doubt permeated my being, and I took cold comfort from sharing the authors' thinly veiled anxiety.

Moreover, as I read these authors, my life was coming to resemble that of the narrators. By day I sat in my armchair, lost in the imaginary creations of Stendhal or Sterne or Beckett. I perceived the campus life around me as through a sheet of cellophane, observing changes in seasons, undergraduates coming and going with each class hour, each semester, each school year. A series of housemates enrolled in shorter programs came, studied, graduated, and moved on. Everyone else seemed to be pursuing specific paths, consciously shaping their lives through actions programmed into their internal hard drives. My actions in the world, including my interactions with others, on the other hand, always seemed somehow misguided, or at best ineffectual. All I knew how to do was think.

And so the days, and months, passed. But it is the nights I remember most vividly. For as long as I sat in the library, I could distract myself with the pantheon of writers arrayed on various syllabi. There was always something to be read. At night I was left to myself, to the endless perambulations of my own mind. The quieter my external life became, the more limited my contact with others, the more agitated my thoughts.

I have always had trouble sleeping. Even as I child, I would toss and turn, disturbed by fears that the house would burn down during the night or that I had forgotten to do my home-work. But my insomnia fully blossomed in the Princeton years, when, without the constraints of regular employment, the pre-dictable rhythms of family life, or any other externally imposed schedule, I slipped into a nocturnal routine of my own devising. I slept all morning, having trained housemates and family not to disturb me before 11:00. Library work began around midday and continued until closing time (11:30 P.M.), when I would cross the street to the town bar to drink with friends until they closed down. On weekends I often stayed up all night and slept through the day. None of this struck me as odd; nor did it occur to me that *I* was becoming odd.

But I did know that I was having more and more trouble sleep-ing, and that many days passed in the disheveled consciousness of the sleep-deprived. Though my mind was crystal-clear in the wee hours of the night, by day I felt fuzzy and forgetful, unable to sustain attention while reading or writing. I had chronic head-aches around my temples, and my energy rose and crashed like waves of jet lag. My therapist doled out sleeping pills in sets of six, fearful that I would build a chemical dependency. I supple-mented the pharmaceuticals with alcohol and all manner of over-the-counter cold remedies that promised drowsiness.

Therapy proved powerless over my insomnia, so I did what I always did when confronted with a challenge: I turned to my mind for help. In twelve-step phraseology, I tried to fix a sick brain with a sick brain. Specifically, I began reading and writing about the plight of the ever-active mind. Insomnia became the subject of my comparative literature dissertation and of a series of related poems.

First I came up with a psychological model of insomnia. I believe that in my own case I only felt safe when I was awake and alert. I equated being conscious with being in control; thus I strove to maintain what a later therapist described as a state of "hypervigilance." (Therapist Number One once pictured me thus: I am sitting in the cockpit of a 747, never having flown before, as the plane makes a nosedive for the ground. On my lap is the flight manual, and I am trying desperately to learn how to fly before the plane crashes.) But circumstances again and again showed me that I was *not* in control, and from this I concluded that I needed not only to be alert but to be *informed*, to have enough information to know how to act in any given situation. And so began the desperate quest for knowledge, for the sort of knowledge that would protect me. What I really needed was omniscience, a Godlike vision of everything that might transpire, and anyone with a shred of spiritual awareness would at that point have headed for the temple or the mosque, the church or the ashram, head bowed in humility before the complexity of Creation. But that only came later. At the time I still thought it was up to me to protect me, to guide me.

And so, from grade school through graduate school and beyond, I had been collecting information. I cast my net wide, studying advanced mathematics, philosophy, languages and literature, history and the social sciences. I kept looking for the master key that would make sense of the mystery, diminish the unknown, bring the darkness into light. I think of the title of a novel by Georges Perec: *Life: A User's Manual.* If the manual didn't exist (and I never really thought it did), I would write my own, culled from the wisdom I had so tirelessly gathered. And then I would fall asleep.

> While looking for the answer, or the answers, to a given question, I
> found the answer, or the answers to a question I had already asked
> myself in vain, in the sense that I had not been able to answer it, or I
> found another question, or other questions, demanding in their turn
> an immediate answer.
>
> —Samuel Beckett, *Molloy*

> What can you expect, they don't know who they are either, nor
> where they are, nor what they're doing. So they build up hypothe-
> ses that collapse on top of one another, it's human, a lobster couldn't
> do it.
>
> —Samuel Beckett, *The Unnamable*

But I could never get "enough" knowledge. Books were taking
over my time and my space, crowding the room where I tried to
sleep in that pastoral New Jersey "bedroom" community. I
bought books before clothes or food. Never satisfied, my mind
absorbed each new theory, each worldview, each hypothesis,
only to reject each in turn as unsatisfactory, inadequate, fatally.
Yet my restless mind went on, and hence the second characteris-
tic of insomnia: The mind is constantly propelled without actually progressing along any linear path, agitated by what are in
Sanskrit referred to as vrttis, disturbances of the field of consciousness.

> It's not a question of hypotheses, it's a question of going on, it goes
> on, hypotheses are like everything else, they help you on.
>
> —Samuel Beckett, *The Unnamable*

The more I thought, the less I knew. Everything began to seem
arbitrary. Although upon finishing graduate school I supported
myself as a critic, I gradually lost the courage of my convictions.
Not that I thought my ideas and opinions were wrong; rather I
just became aware that they were merely ideas and opinions and
that their relationship to "reality," to the texts or artworks they
attempted to evaluate, were at best arbitrary, even accidental. In
the poststructuralist view (which, I later discovered, shares
much with Buddhist psychology), what I call "I" is merely a collection of codes, of contingencies that arise in such a way as to

make "me" experience (and perceive) things in a certain way at a certain moment. Given the circumstantial and highly individualistic nature of perception, it dawned on me that my opinions were probably not of much use to anyone else, and that they might in fact be causing some inadvertent harm. (Careers are often shaped by the words of influential critics, and I had become a functioning cog in this machinery.) Sometime thereafter I sent out postcards to everyone I knew announcing: "For one day, February 29, I will utter no words of judgment. This anomalous date (which occurs only in leap years), struck me as an appropriate time for anomalous behavior. Since I make my living as a critic, I am constantly passing judgments."

This "behavior piece," as I called it, an early item in my series of conceptual art projects, effectively marked the beginning of the end of my life as a critic. Entitled *Too Many Critics*, it reflected my sinking sense of the futility of the critical genre.

Giving up my career was a lot easier than facing the underlying identity crisis. I had always identified myself with my ideas, with my opinions, with my likes and dislikes and my ability to justify them. I *was* this constellation of hard-won views, collected and stored on the hard drive of my mind. As this seemingly firm infrastructure began to waiver and shift, I lost my bearings. I was becoming fluid, insubstantial, protean, while everyone around me seemed to remain solid, substantial, settled.

> But where has art led us? . . . It has cast us out of our power to begin and to end; it has turned us toward the outside where there is no intimacy and no place to rest. It has led us into the infinite migration of error.
> —Maurice Blanchot, quoted in Mark C. Taylor, "Descartes, Nietzsche, and the Search for the Unsayable," *New York Times Book Review*, 1 February 1987: 34.

> These fragments I have shored against my ruins . . . .
> —T. S. Eliot, *The Waste Land*

Every instinct was telling me to hide, to go "underground," to withdraw physically to protect what was left of my disintegrating self. Proust did it, and Beckett after him, and I had all those fictional models of withdrawal arrayed on my bookshelves. I would be in good company in my isolation. I would find my home among the insomniacs, the weirdos, the misfits. But some part of me resisted, some part would not go silent into that dark night.

Instead, I began producing artworks that indirectly reflected my plight. A series entitled *Home/Homesick/Homeless* ostensibly began as a scrutiny of New York City's homeless crisis but rapidly broadened into an inquiry into the notion of "home." That I felt some strong identification with the homeless, alienated and adrift, emerged in a behavior piece in which for the month of January I wore only clothes collected off the streets. In *Homesick Photos* I went around the city photographing other people's apartments, documenting how other people created a (physical) sense of home, looking for clues to what might make an "appropriate" shell for my floundering self. I also photographed my own place, and with the eerie detachment enforced by the camera lens, I studied my so-called home like a pathologist scrutinizing a deviant cell. What was missing? How come my place never felt like home?

For a New York project entitled *Trespassing*, I made a list of all the places in the city (neighborhoods, public spaces, private clubs and institutions, types of businesses) where I cannot, may not, or should not go. Then I went to those places and recorded what happened. At some point along the way the list of places grew so long that I felt compelled to list places I *did* belong. It was woefully short, and for each item on the list I could conjure up some reason why I didn't quite belong there either.

> I contradict myself? Very well then, I contradict myself. I am vast. I contain multitudes.
>
> —Walt Whitman, "Song of Myself"

It was while working on these pieces that I had my "spiritual awakening." I like to think that God, or fate, or karma, or whatever power governs the material plane took me right to my edge before lifting the veil of doubt and confusion. Actually, I'm still confused most of the time, at least whenever I try to wrap my mind around the nature of any Supreme Power. While rereading *The Yoga Sutras* the other day, I caught myself debating whether I believe in Patanjali's purusha (true self) or whether I subscribe to the Buddhist view that there is no self. Or did I think it was okay to believe in both, to contradict myself? Or to somehow encompass both? Or to never really know? In other words, I caught myself once again *forming an opinion,* trying to settle things once and for all. I recalled the words of a wise friend who once advised: "Seek the seekers of the Truth, and run from those who have found it."

But yoga for the most part saves me from abstract speculation by keeping me busy with *practices*: asanas, pranayama, chanting, meditation. And the more I practice, the less I need to speculate. The more I practice, the more I stay tuned to my experience, and experiences are gradually coming to replace opinions in my mind. I find, in line with vipassana, that I can watch ideas, concepts, opinions arise and fall away with each passing moment—especially the concept of my so-called self that gave me so much trouble earlier on.

The internal redirection began with that New York yoga class. By all accounts I felt alienated in that East Village studio: the purple walls, the incense and altars, the Sanskrit chanting. A Modernist and minimalist, I prefer blank white walls, fresh air, and silence. Yet as I started to move through the postures, bending and breathing and basically just trying to keep up (the class moved in a rapid vinyassa style that was totally new to me), I got my second message from above. Again, it was admirably simple:

Welcome home.

I felt that I was meant to be doing these postures, that I was *designed* to do them. I left class feeling pliable yet strong, with a resilience that made life's challenges less threatening. I no longer felt "a short distance from my body"; for once my mind connected to my bones, and I looked out of eyes attached to my head. And somehow I sensed (I am reluctant anymore to say that I "knew" or know anything) that I was on the path to peace. Enlightenment was too lofty a concept for me then, and still is; I just wanted the anguish to end. And for the most part it has.

I am not my body; I am not my mind.

So we chanted during one of my early yoga classes. What a relief! I need no longer identify with my mind or my body. Still, I am left on the material plane with both a body and a mind, and both continue to test my spirit. A few years into my yoga practice I went to India to study Ashtanga yoga under Sri K. Pattabhi Jois. I carried home an abundance of parasites, some of which I apparently still host. My health went downhill fast, as my weakened immune system succumbed to various secondary infections. Looking back, I see that years of poor nutrition and compulsive activity had pushed my system to the verge of collapse. India—or perhaps contact with the compassionate yet penetrating gaze of my guru—merely brought the truth to the surface.

And so began my physical reeducation. I learned to cook. I learned to eat. I learned more about the body (and my body in particular) than I had ever cared to. I learned that asking for help and accepting the myriad forms (well meaning but misguided, direct but unpalatable, informed yet impenetrable, costly in all cases) in which it is offered by doctors, therapists, and healers is itself a spiritual practice.

Meanwhile, my Ashtanga practice has stagnated, backpedaled, inched forward, slid back, and blossomed so many times that I have jettisoned the notion of "progress" so dear to my Western conditioning. When I was too sick even to sit for meditation, I settled into the healing grace of restorative yoga and deep sleep. When you can't walk, crawling looks great. When you can't sit, lying down will do. I suspect that the amoebae still lodged in my gut will stay with me until I have fully absorbed the lesson of self-care.

As for the mind, my thoughts still keep me up many a night, but now I play with mantras, watch my breath, say prayers. And while calming habitually tense nerves may be a lifetime project, I no longer despair that I am condemned to sleepless vigilance. Whatever the nature of "I" may be, I no longer believe that "I" am in charge.

Buddhism teaches that the fixed self is a delusion created by the frightened ego and that each moment of experience arises out of ever-changing conditions. As Heraclitus pointed out centuries ago, I cannot step into the same river twice because "I" am never the same. I do not exist independent of time and circumstance.

The more I clung to my disappearing self, the more isolated and alienated I felt. While this is a spiritual truism in some circles, I had to experience it over months and years before I surrendered my grip. (I still struggle with the labels I pin on myself, which cramp my style and stifle my spirit.) Throughout it all, and through some act of grace, yoga offers me glimpses of the other side, of life *not* focused on the isolated self.

> Only connect.
>
> —E. M. Forster, *Howards End*

Connecting internally—coming home—has also made it possible for me to connect with others. With the help of friends, yogis, and a spiritually grounded career counselor, I gathered the courage to abandon my old life and devote myself to practicing and teaching yoga. Teaching has been the greatest gift, for when I immerse myself in sharing yoga with others, all our separate selves seem to dissolve, or at least to lose their sharp edges. Swami Vivekananda wrote that the definition of love is "pure attention." When I can give that to my students, "I" feel connected to them and to everything that is.

journey in yama-yama land
Robert Perkins

> Depression is the reward you get for being good.
> — Marion Woodman, *Addicted to Perfection*

I like a little space around me, a little solitude. I've been in the Arctic three weeks, and for me, that's just warming up. There are several hundred miles between myself and the next human being, not to mention the nearest town. There's more sky here than anything else, unless it's water, or silence. I've always been a water rat: My best strength is to be like water.

I'm on a big, beautiful, northern river. I've been on it before. It flows uninterrupted for six hundred miles to the Arctic Ocean. Take out a map of Canada, locate the Great Slave Lake in the

There is no direct connection between the title of this essay and the yoga yamas. The title came to me after a yoga class during deep relaxation, unbidden. I knew nothing of the yoga yamas, or laws, then.

Northwest Territory, then run your finger in a northeasterly direction until you find the thin blue line of the Back River. When my friends ask me where I'm off to, and I tell them, they say, "Back to the Back, eh?" And I smile, and say to myself, yes, back to the Back. I no longer explain or justify my trips. I have not heard a motor for three weeks, or seen another person. (That is not exactly true. Once a week I hear the slightest automated rumble high up, 33,000 feet high up, as I watch the white contrail of a jet spread across the blue, blue sky.)

Last night, the caribou came at eleven P.M. They woke me up. I lay there listening to them belch, fart, and huff before I saw them. Thousands of them were across the river running a ridge, silhouetted against an orange sherbet sunset. Because they were silhouettes, they looked flat, like noisy paper cutouts. I was half asleep as I watched the caribou. I remembered, as a child, moving small metal toys over a piece of paper by sliding a magnet around underneath. Maybe because of that, or because it was twilight and their dark silhouettes made the caribou look flat, as flat and same-colored as the ridge they traveled over, they seemed to be connected to the ridge, more like part of the earth getting up to move around than separate things. The caribou were all sizes, a huge part of the Beverly herd. Big bulls moved forward bobbing their racks as they crossed the ridge. Mothers doubled back looking for their calves. Calves bleated mournfully for their mothers. Young bucks pranced, throwing their heads–all in silhouette.

Then they were swarming around my tent. The caribou's ankle joints make an odd clicking sound as they move. It's a tendon sliding across bone that makes the clicking. The Inuit call caribou *tuck-tu* after this sound. I carefully unzipped the mosquito netting so that I could see better. At times there were only legs in front of the tent, or a head would dip down, snatch at a tuft of grass, and keep moving. A constant restlessness. There had been a field of lupine in bloom around me. In the morning, there were only a few that hadn't been trampled or eaten.

Then they were gone. The eerie thing was the silence that poured back in. An intense stillness returned, and the tundra seemed to fall back into its waitingness. A small sparrow, a lark-spur, called from somewhere far off, punctuating the stillness with its prestissimo. I lay in the tent listening, dazed by what in the morning seemed more a dream than something that had really happened.

Yama-Yama Land is my name for depression's terrain. I am not depressed today, but my journey in Yama-Yama Land lasted six years. I've never seen the land written up in an eco-tour guide, and you can't find it on a map. It's an expensive place to visit (in more ways than one). The journey is both harrowing and really boring, sometimes both at once. You can't describe it to anyone who hasn't been there. Slides don't help. For all their books, but one, the Explorer's Club doesn't mention it. However, Yama-Yama Land is real, the way the Terra Incognita drawn onto the old maps was real—it has a place in the world, yet no one knows much about it. If issued a ticket, it's hard not to go. But to survive the journey takes courage. Simply put, Yama-Yama Land sucks.

I remember exactly when I entered Yama-Yama Land, but I am hard pressed to say, as clearly, when I returned. My journey began the evening of August 17, 1994, the day my wife of four months died. Rene had been fighting breast cancer, then the awful effects of its cure, for two and a half years. We married that April, thinking she would be stable. If we made it to five years, we might see ten. Why not? Many others had. In June her vision blurred. They found tiny tumors in her eyes. Her constant cough turned into difficult breathing. Her lungs ossified. In August, she died.

Several times during my six years in Yama-Yama Land, I came north alone to canoe. Twice, I could have killed myself. Before entering Yama-Yama Land and losing Rene, I had no concept of afterlife. I never believed in it, but I do now. There is life after death, but not the way I imagined. It is not a churchy thing. After-life is what happens to us here, to me. It is literally that: after life. I entered it the night Rene died. It was my passport to Yama-Yama Land. In it, I wandered like smoke, floated there, blown any which way for all those years.

At the worst point in the journey (which was pretty much the whole time), I could not have written about yoga and depression. But I am back now. And I must tell you something of what happened, how yoga played its part. The words I'll use are dry and linear, time bound, and guaranteed to release, if at all, merely an echo, or an aroma, of what Yama-Yama Land is truly like. Our language isn't great at conveying the "verb" state of things. Neither yoga nor depression is easily put into words. Both yoga and depression are organic, lusciously so, and work in and out of time. They are not verbal.

My fall into depression was more like Coyote's run off the cliff in the *Road Runner* cartoons than the graceful, arcing dive of a swimmer. When Coyote misses the Road Runner he pauses for a moment, graced by the cartoonist with enough time to look down and realize he's about to fall. Then the perspective shifts. We watch from above, Coyote's round eyes looking up at us as he falls. The sound of a low whistle accompanies him down. A small dust cloud rises when he hits bottom. I prefer this humorous way of imagining my entry into Yama-Yama Land. In reality, I went over the cliff badly, hardly knowing I had left solid ground. I had no cartoonist to draw for me. I had to find it all out for myself.

I would talk with a psychiatrist, William Ackerly. He would nod his head in agreement and say, "Yes, Rob, it *is* awful. Yes, it *is* terrible." When he would say this he would look down and to the left. He never told me what was wrong with me. He never disagreed with me the way friends or family would, admonishing me to snap out of "it," or worse, assume "it" had passed.

What I value most is what he did concerning medication. My internist is a young doctor, who simply said, "Look, Rob. When you break a leg, you get a cast. When you get a cut, you put a Band-Aid on it. So, you're depressed. You are in pain. Why not take a designer drug like Zoloft or Prozac? You don't have to suffer." I was tempted, sorely tempted. In Yama-Yama Land you grab at what relief is offered, be it food, sex, drugs, alcohol, even suicide. In response to my desire to take the medication, Ackerly always asked a question. He would sit there opposite me and listen to how awful it felt. He'd say he'd write the prescription, if that was what I really wanted. Then he'd ask me, as though he hadn't heard my request, "And what medication does your internist want to offer a man whose soul has been ripped in half? Why wouldn't you be in pain?" I did not take the medication and feel I won a slightly more secure victory for having weathered my depression without drugs.

I grew up coddled in a middle-class world. One of that world's tenets is to be polite. The good side of being polite is that you overlook things. The bad side of being polite is that you overlook things. You're either being considerate of others, or, if you are too well mannered, you are truly "overlooking." If you don't notice long enough, you become disconnected. You know neither what's really happening inside you, what feelings you are having, or what's happening in the larger world. You unplug. After long enough, you don't even know you're unplugged. Instead of listening carefully to your best advisor (your body), you ignore it.

My model was my dad. I never knew what he was feeling. I never knew what he was thinking, and after I went away to boarding school, I had even less chance of ever knowing. He had lived through the depression. He had fought in the Second World War. He flew dive bombers off aircraft carriers in the Pacific. His generation needed to ignore their feelings. But at what cost, I wonder.

I was brought up to "do" things with my body: run with a football, tackle people, hit a tennis ball, paddle a canoe, cast a fly-line. The idea of becoming conscious about what my body was actually doing *while* I was "doing" was a revelation. This is what my yoga practice has given me. The realization that I breathe, that tension and anxiety have their roots in the mind and their blossom in the body; that the body itself is such an amazing instrument all on its own (let alone what you can do with it)—all this was a sobering revelation. Certainly it was a departure from anything my home life, or schooling, prepared me for.

Yoga was counterculture in the 1960s. I was twenty. I was a good athlete, captain of my high school football team, goalie on the hockey team, and New England School Boy pole vault champ (for about a week) at the height of 13 feet, 5 inches. Try as I could, and I tried, I could not get that next quarter-inch. At Harvard College, I decided I did not want to be competitive anymore. I went looking for something else. That's when I encountered yoga. There was a hectic, free-wheeling, three-hour class held twice a week, open to anyone, at any skill level, at the Unitarian church, Zero Church Street in Cambridge. Bingo. I was hooked. I was there every week. The teacher, John Loder, was a handsome man who looked like Peter O'Toole in *Lawrence of Arabia.* Many evenings I had to elbow my way through all the beautiful women to find mat space up front near him. I was there to learn as much as I could. The women were up front to learn as much as they could, too. I guess. I was one of the few men in the class. There must be an unwritten rule that women in yoga classes (especially pretty ones) don't talk to men unless you are the instructor. At least, I've never had a conversation with a woman that lasted more than thirty seconds.

John taught hatha yoga. He would demonstrate a move, then go into the movement's repetitions and combinations. There were often seventy-five to a hundred people in the room. We followed as best we could. More advanced students tried to keep people from hurting themselves, or toppling into others. I broke a woman's nose when I fell out of a headstand, but most of the time, people survived and enjoyed themselves. After several years, the class stopped. I did, too.

During my early twenties, I went back to my high school to teach yoga for a term. My high point came after lunch, demonstrating a headstand in the faculty room to all the fuddy-duddy teachers who had taught me. My old English teacher, A. O. Smith, remarked under his breath, but loud enough for me to hear him: "There are many ways to get your feet off the ground. I prefer my way–it's called a vodka martini."

I have to explain my body. It is not flexible or supple. It has too much muscle to do half the postures, or asanas, correctly. More easily, I can hold positions that take strength. There is a man in the class I attend, Neal, who is as good as any woman. He has hip joints like butter, and strength and grace and balance. I know we're all working on our own bodies, at our own speed, but what I wouldn't give for half of Neal's flexibility and grace.

In the 1970s, I read the books, especially Krishnamurti. I wasn't as bad as Jackson Pollock in his twenties, who was so taken with Krishnamurti that he began dressing like him, but I was bad enough. All day long I spouted Eastern wisdomisms to family and friends. I sought the death of my ego and the clutter that had collected around it. In my twenties, my desire was to get away from myself, from my problems, to forget. Now I realize that's not any informed yoga student's goal. It led me nowhere. It might be fair to say that it kept me from dealing with my particular life. Or did it? I don't really know.

Eventually, life pushed me in other directions. It was twenty years before I began to practice yoga again. This time I entered through another door. Do people make life changes, I wonder, if they're not forced into them?

Today, I caught two lake trout. The trout in the Arctic are not difficult to catch. They're hungry. I fished from the canoe as I drifted through fast water at the foot of a rapid. Three casts, two fish. I don't need a net to get them in the canoe. I used my spinning rod, and a red-and-white Dar-Devil lure, and a long steel leader. I pull them out of the water by the steel leader. In the canoe I hit them on the head, or bend their necks back until they break. I put the fish in a plastic bag to avoid having fish smell on my canoe or on my pants. Bears are attracted to the smell of fish. The one thing I don't want is to meet a Barren Grounds grizzly bear at close quarters. I've accepted the possibility that I might die out here, but I am not happy with the thought of dying *slowly* out here.

Before I sat down to begin writing tonight, I cooked the trout over an open fire. I had found the top of a ten-inch grill at an earlier campsite. I laid the fish, one at a time, on the grill, split open, skin side down. Before cooking them, I rubbed olive oil and sprinkled salt and pepper on them. The skin against the flames kept the flesh from burning. I ate their lovely, pink flesh with my fingers.

Rene's breast cancer led her, and myself, into the world of alternative healing. Her decision was to do Western medicine and alternative therapies, and hope for the best. She became a macrobiotic eater. I did, too, except when I headed out to Bartley's Burger Cottage or a steak house (with Rene's blessing). We tried many therapies. We went to a small town in Switzerland to the Rudolph Steiner Cancer Clinic for Rene to receive injections of mistletoe. I can feel the heavy silence of the clinic cafeteria where I would join her for lunch. Conversation at meals was not encouraged. I still can hear the lonely clinks of those oversized silver spoons in the soup bowls. A journey in Yama-Yama Land takes you to many different places.

Our habits, our patterns, and our securities became unbuttoned one by one until, sadly, Rene was left holding only pain—and the knowledge that she was deeply loved by her family, her friends, and by me. She knew, too, that she would die.

An early therapy was to go on a macrobiotic/yoga retreat. I'm a New Englander, a Baked Bean. We rely on ourselves. We're stoics. The New England coastline isn't made of granite for nothing. It takes a long time to wear down a good piece of granite, or a cold-roast New Englander. By nature, we're not fuzzy, touchy-feely, group-oriented people. I went reluctantly to the retreat. At the time, "retreat" sounded just like that, "a going away from," a retreat.

Karin Stephan ran the retreat. There were several other couples, one each of whom had an illness. She tolerated those like me, and worked compassionately with the others. I intuited, more than I realized, that she was a healer. Back in Boston, Rene and I occasionally attended macrobiotic dinners at her loft or dropped in on a yoga class.

By the February after Rene's death, I had ground to a halt. On the outside I didn't look any different, but I was a wreck. I couldn't sleep. My enthusiasm evaporated. I had no appetite. I drank too much. I ate a lot of Spam. For a year, the only consistent thing I did was see Bill Ackerly. I had crossed the border into Yama-Yama Land and I had no clue how to get out.

I saw Karin on the street in Cambridge. She reminded me that she held yoga classes in her loft three evenings a week. Like a

ghost, I began to attend her Wednesday evening class, sporadi-
cally and without conviction. Karin mentioned that she taught
private lessons. I began to come to her loft in the afternoons,
occasionally. More often, I'd make an appointment and never
show up.

That's what I mean when I say a journey in Yama-Yama Land
is expensive. During these years, I not only spent money without
making any, I also lost friends and the respect of others, including my respect for myself. I had no capacity to engage. A
frustration for me was that I knew all this about myself. I knew I
was unhappy. What I didn't know was how to change it.

On my canoe trips, I bring a pink flamingo, the plastic kind
people stick in their front lawns for decoration. I use it for a lawn
decoration, too. Being alone, I'm my own entertainment, and
walking back to camp, seeing my flamingo, makes me smile.
This summer I saw something new in Yellowknife—rows of alternating red and yellow plastic tulips, five to a strip. I bought a strip
and substituted them for the flamingo. The ground squirrels, or
sic-sics, play with them.

During one of the two summers I could have killed myself, I
sat on a knoll on a gray day, hood up. Quiet and still, I looked
inland. Sometimes I'll sit like that for an hour, challenging
myself to see new things. The tundra is huge and flat like the
ocean. Its colors are sharper on a dull day. They stand out more.
That day, in the distance, I saw something white. I guessed it was
a seagull flying low over the land hoping to flush some small
creature. The bird was flying in my general direction. As it came
closer, I could see it was not a seagull, but a snowy owl. I held my
breath. It flew right at me, missing my head by only three feet. As
it passed, it turned its head and gave me a deep, long look. I heard
nothing. Its wings gave no sound. I watched it fly its zigzag
course low over the ground, back and forth slowly, thoughtfully,
until it became a salt grain, then disappeared, and I was left sitting there, wondering if it had happened at all.

When Karin started working with me, we didn't know each
other. Over the next four years, we came to know each other well.
She told me how, when she met me on the street, she saw a shell

around me. That first year and a half, she knew I was protecting myself like a mollusk, and all she could initially give me was a safe place to come. She was always optimistic and strong. What she didn't know was whether I'd keep coming back. She didn't care how long we had to wait. Her goal was to activate my energy; get me to move. We did asanas that would stimulate my adrenal glands and kidneys: backbends, and inversions. Twists would have been good, but my body does not twist easily. Standing on my head, or the shoulderstand, was easier.

Those first months, we spoke very little. She's told me since then she knew that talking would do no good. Being mostly silent allowed her to tune into my body. On days when I kept our appointments, I remember the warmth of her loft, her soft voice and offhand manner. Often, I came in the afternoon when the light streamed in her west-facing windows. I had no energy. I would lie in that light, softly crying. Occasionally, she could get me to work on my body a little. Then, I'd leave, feeling no better, seeing no change. But I kept returning.

Later, Karin told me something about her own journey in Yama-Yama Land. When she began working with me, she said, the feeling that surfaced was when she had felt like lead herself. The image for her was walking with her dad along the shore of Lake Champlain in Vermont. This was near the end of his life. He was old, and she was in her late thirties, yet he was pulling her as a child would pull a wagon.

She would say to him, "Dad, I can't walk anymore. I'm tired."

He would insist in the most loving way, "No, you must walk." He knew he had to keep her moving. Because of this, the day that Karin met me on the street, she knew where I was.

As we became friends, Karin told me how her commitment to yoga had begun. In 1969, she studied yoga in Paris with Jean Bennard Rishi. She traveled with him and six others to India to visit a little-known yogi called Pattabhi Jois. He was an English-speaking yogi and Karin's job was to translate his lectures on the Bhagavad Gita for the Frenchmen.

While she was in India, she met Krishnamurti. She sat in on lectures he gave about dying to the moment. She remembers him saying something that made no sense to her then. "Prepare for death in life by dying to each moment." Even though she didn't understand everything happening to her in India, she felt she had come home. Karin was twenty-seven.

But it was a side visit that unexpectedly transformed her life. She was along for the ride to visit the French colony called Pondicherry. Her friend wanted to visit an ashram in the colony and pay his respects to a spiritual teacher known as The Mother. She was ninety-four years old. An hour outside Pondicherry, the bus broke down. While waiting for the bus to get fixed, Karin felt a huge sense of peace flood her body. She felt a oneness with everything, serene, as though she'd been embraced. These were feelings she had never had before. She didn't know it then, but she understood later that she had received a benediction.

At the moment Karin felt flooded with peace and love, The Mother was giving darshan. *Darshan* means "to see." The Mother had come out on a balcony to gaze at her disciples. Karin says it is a silent thing. There's no talking, no lecture, no teaching, just presence, pure presence. And Karin received her benediction an hour away, sitting in a broken-down bus. I asked her if there was anything else specific that she could remember. She became shy and only said she would never forget that her benediction happened in 1969 on November 21, at 8 P.M.

Thanks to a disciple of Gandhi, Major Rama Chandra, Karin had a personal darshan with The Mother. She sat in front of Mother, looking in her eyes. They held a silent conversation. Then, Mother gave her a rose, the color of which tells you what you need to work on in your life. Karin got a yellow rose. That meant Karin lived too much on the mental plane—that she would have to break away from the mental process as a means of perceiving reality. I wonder if I didn't receive something similar to darshan the day I sat on that rock and the snowy owl flew by. I didn't know it then but the owl's closeness, and those yellow eyes, held me.

She initially studied with Pattabhi Jois, who she remembers had incredible hands, big strong hands, deft at adjusting your position, but she shifted to follow Iyengar because he was, as she says, "so sassy and fierce. It was exciting." She remembers once being in a shoulderstand on a cement floor in a lotus position. Iyengar gently pushed her knees on the floor to either side of her head. He grunted and said, "No one has ever made you to do this before, huh?" She took it as an invitation to push herself. When Iyengar first came to the West, to London, Paris, and Amsterdam, Karin traveled with him.

In 1976, Karin arrived in Boston. Before moving to Cambridge, she lived and worked on Beacon Hill. By 1985 she had opened the area's Iyengar Center with another woman who followed Iyengar, Patricia Walden. Karin is interested in yoga as a healing therapy—she feels that Iyengar gave her courage to take on the pain of difficult situations. She works with individuals, like myself, and small groups, "to awaken," as she says, "various aspects of themselves in the field of physical health and balance."

Her way worked for me. Slowly, she saw a growing plasticity in my mind, a fluidity, and my body began to have more energy. My heaviness disappeared. Karin was creative in her combinations, constantly changing them as she received information from me on many levels, what I was resisting as well as what I was willing to let in. She works in the living presence, the "now" of the person. She likes quoting a Rumi poem: "When angels achieved discipline, they began to shine."

In the Arctic, I watch the wind. On a calm night, like tonight, there's a little wind, a soft breath, that crosses over the face of the water just after sunset, a moment of balance between the day's many forces. Nature is very quiet, isn't she? Why, tonight, it's grown dark, the sun has set. The moon is out. The colors of the red spectrum splashed across the clouds, and not one sound did I hear through the whole extraordinary performance. They say it's even quieter in outer space, utterly silent. I wouldn't know—and I wouldn't care to know about that silence. Equally to silence I love the wind that brings me sounds: the buzz of the bugs, the rumble of a rapid, the single call of a bird, or many birds. Sometimes the wind can hide things, too, smells and sounds. Sometimes, the wind is bossy, pushing hard on everything, ruthless with anything weakly attached: a broken branch, a tent, a leaf, a loose canoe. It plays with water, sometimes stroking it, other times beating it like a hand whips egg whites. It brings in the clouds and dusts them away. And you never see it, except through what it touches. It's a mystery, a medium. It's where spirit lives.

Life is breath, isn't it? Slow cycles of in and out: breathing, day turning into night, summer into winter, our life into another life, in loving, in dying. We say hello. We say good-bye. We say hello again. The older Inuit knew the European Christians who came to the North had only part of the story. It's not only the soul that's immortal. The Inuit could see the body was immortal, too. They saw this around them—everything eaten, transformed into something else. Each thing itself eventually transformed, even the earth, but always part of, and connected to, the rest of life. Where something dies, greener grass grows. But I like the wind, the way it comes in close, tussles my paper, tugs at the edge of my anorak's hood. On my first trips, I never gave the wind a thought. Yes, I'd check to see if it was a head wind, or not, but if someone had told me the wind had a voice, I would have laughed. After twenty years of traveling here, I know the wind has a voice, and a huge vocabulary. It constantly speaks. If we don't listen, that's OK. It passes on like a letter unopened. But I know what it says now. Like an annunciation, it whispers in my ear, "Surprise me."

the art of breathing

Reetika Vazirani

Europe discovers. India beckons. Isn't that so? India sits atop her lily pad through centuries, lost in contemplation of the horizon. And, from time to time, India is discovered.

—Richard Rodriguez, *Days of Obligation*

"What's she do all day, stranded on top of that cliff?"

"She curls up with the *Upanishads*. She's been reading the *Upanishads* in paperback for the last three years. She feels the East is where truth is, what she calls the petal of all energy. Non-attachment turns her on."

—Don DeLillo, *Great Jones Street*

1. Atlantic Coast Athletic Club

My yoga instructor, Jennifer, is a white woman from Virginia. She studied Ashtanga yoga with one of its founders, K. Pattabhi Jois in Mysore, India, and with Jois's disciple Richard Freeman in Colorado. I am the only East Indian in the class; everybody else is white and American born. This becomes most apparent to me every time the class mispronounces the Sanskrit names for particular asanas. This has been going on for nearly two years. When the class mispronounces *Surya Namaskara,* sun salutation, I feel a murmur of discomfort, the way I feel today in my obstetrician's office when my own name is mangled. Calling me for my ultrasound, the receptionist leans towards the glass window, Retinka Varzeenee. How can this be? I have been here once a month for seven months and have corrected her four times.

How do the vowels of *Surya Namaskara* become "saryee nemiskra"? I associate the butchering of sound first with the British who took the city Kul-kutta and said "Cal-cut'-a"; Joe-dh-poor, the name of the city, became "jod-per," the horseback-riding breeches. Could the impulse behind drastically changing a word's original sound have something to do with the newcomer's wish to take the word away from its source and personalize it? Perhaps to extract the word from its culture and to co-opt it? I am talking about mispronunciation which goes far beyond the newcomer's inability to make certain sounds. *Surya* spoken by an American speaker need not become "saryee," any more than *sun* needs to become "sin" or "soon" in Hindi. Even after a year of following along with our instructor, the class will not come closer to the original Sanskrit pronunciations. To me, the privilege of not taking the time to say a word or name correctly has something to do with a First World country borrowing from a southern nation-state. It is part of the (benign?) entitlement deployed by a culturally curious, ardent, and even visionary sector of America's leisure class. The lazy pronunciation signals part of the removal of yoga from its Sanskrit sources, meanings, aspirations, and a movement towards pure workout; or, as Ashtanga yoga is often labeled, power yoga.

I am reminded of *patchouli, khaki, gyro, chimichanga, sushi, gewürztraminer, gharam masala, dungarees* on a menu at the all-night deli counter and flea market of Creole that is the English dictionary, that book of migration and immigration from which I take citizenship. I imagine I am the only person in the class who can properly pronounce most of the Sanskrit words. But, like the other participants, I need a translator, Jennifer.

After two years, I have to stop practicing yoga in Jennifer's Ashtanga classes, because the routine (the primary series) is too strenuous for pregnant women. I cannot do the twists and backbends. I rely on breathing techniques I learned from her.

When I first learn to practice ujjayi breathing–when I close off part of the back of my throat and begin to breath with a meditative hum to my inhalations and exhalations–I begin to generate heat in my body.

The heat in my body leads me to spaces within myself, as if to rooms in a house I had never let myself fully inhabit. I can enter deep and secret rooms, light and dark rooms–spaces between my vertebrae and the warm pouch of my pancreas. These spaces take on a kind of cleansing, and I begin to feel the intimacy of the freedom of my breath.

When I stop competing with others over how flexible or strong I would like to be, I begin to notice my breath threading into my capillaries. My perineum wakes, and I learn to suck air from the center of the earth. I learn to exhale through the top of my head, and the new tingling in my fingers pulses with the shimmer and strength I feel in my perineum.

Yoga is a discipline of tenderness for and awareness of the body–heart, lungs, kidney, pressure points to the inner life of the eye, third eye, eye of the spleen.

The heat generated by my audible breathing leads me underground and overseas.

2. Puja Closet, Maryland

My father comes to America in the fifties to study oral surgery. He returns in 1969, to teach at a university, to begin a private practice, and to join his wife and children who arrived eighteen months before. America wants trained doctors. I learn that my father can also give anesthesia, prescribe painkillers and other drugs. In the midst of the civil rights movement, we Asians enter, and he comes with certain skills.

The university where my father teaches is African-American. His colleagues are dentists and surgeons. I notice that they seem very rich and stylish, and in them resides a certain power, a glamour I am not a part of. This has less to do with the fine clothes they wear. It has to do with voices. Voices and perfumes and colognes. I would like nothing better than to be Mrs. Jeffries, the woman who can make people stop in their tracks as she enters our door. She is head of nursing. To me, she is like Roberta Flack. I am intoxicated and full of admiration for a drama I do not understand.

My elementary school is largely white. When it rains, we have recess indoors. We throw a firm rubber ball to each other. This is called silent speedball. If you drop the ball, you are out. I am usually one of the first to drop the ball, because when it speeds at me, I feel the slap and sting even before I touch it. The ball bruises my knuckles. When it isn't raining, we go outside to recess, and I watch my classmates turn loops on the monkey bars. I marvel at what my classmates can do with their strong bodies. A certain toughness resides in these people, and I am not a part of it, the it which I think of as America–sports, being number one. The white kids in my school are speedy and strong with their bodies, but I cannot seem to make a meaning out of them or a place for myself with them.

Once a week, our house turns Indian. On Thursday evenings, my father lights thin sticks of incense, agarbati, in a shrine he had assembled in my brother's bedroom closet, and we begin our weekly puja, worship service.

This shrine honors my father's two gurus in India. The younger one, about fifty, stands in a black-and-white photo, framed in a simple black wooden frame about thirty by twenty-five inches, on top of the older guru's photo of the same size. The younger guru's large Afro blooms over the long silk stalk of a kurta, (tunic) on which you can still see straight creases from careful ironing. The older guru, perhaps eighty, died a long time ago. He wears a simple cotton scarf over what seems to be a bald head, no shirt, around his waist several layers of cotton cloth. I am told the younger guru, found auspiciously in a village, is the reincarnation of the older. The younger guru looks African-American. The older one looks Cuban or Israeli, or North African; he could be from anywhere. It is not surprising that they are related, for even in my own family there are lighter- and darker-skinned members. And when I sit among this group, I am aware of our variety, and of our blendings between the lighter-skinned people of my father's side, Sindhis, and the darker skins of my mother's side, Bengalis. When I think of the younger guru's Afro, I imagine the days when India hugged the coast of Africa and Madagascar, and all brownness had a central source.

Sprinkled on the floor of the closet around these large photos I see small silver boxes, dishes, wooden incense holders, a silver dish of fruit, sometimes flowers, and photos of some of my father's relatives who died in India. Also, there is a cotton cloth with a checked pattern of deer standing stately by and the word *Welcome* in every square. After five minutes at this temple, I feel uncomfortable. I do not like sitting cross-legged for long periods. In church, my friends sit on hard benches, and I do not like those either. These benches, I learn, are called pews. Why do white people pick the name of a bad smell for their church furniture, I wonder? Why do I associate pews with white people? What is it about discomfort that makes me think of them? All in all, I prefer puja to pews, because when we finish, we just hop downstairs to dinner rather than make our way through a tight chapel doorway to a jammed parking lot where the hair-spray people can run you over. I feel funny: I don't mind seeing white people in church, but right now I would not like white people to see me in puja. What would they say? It is 1970, and they would say we are poor people sitting on the floor. They might even donate some chairs for us. The blue-haired ladies in church shake their affectionate fingers at us, saying we are the clever Vietnamese refugees they are so happy to sponsor.

The worst thing about being Indian, Asian, or brown, is its

association with chronic national poverty, nakedness or tattered clothes, paucity of food, and substandard housing: the feeling that we are under sponsorship, and we are not really who we are, we are who others tell us to be. And, as brown people, we are the quiet recipients of a charity our donors acquired god knows how.

Sitting cross-legged at the foot of our shrine in a closet, I learn how to copy my father's gestures as he repeats his mantra, "Sai Ram," and fingers, one after the other, 108 sandalwood beads on a garland. This he calls "doing mala." I think of all the poor people in the world who have nothing but a string and wooden beads for their worship. I am not aware I am being introduced to yoga, the art of breathing.

On Thursday nights, we sing as a family, led by my father. This is called "doing puja." Afterwards we eat dinner, and I forget there are people in church who think we are poor. Behind me on the wall in the kitchen hangs a Mercator projection of the world, and I know my father travels to Europe to teach doctors how to do surgery. These countries are pale, pink, green, and yellow.

3. Oamkar

During his busy weekdays, before breakfast, my father sits at the closet, inhales, holds his breath, exhales, holds his breath, and says "oam" for as long as he can, over and over. He encourages his children to join him, but I have no memory of the others joining us. My littlest sister is three, my other little sister is six, and my eldest sister has her mind on other things, not oamkar. As for my brother, this is his bedroom, and as I sit with my father at the foot of this closet, I do not know where my brother is. My only memory of this oamkar exercise is of myself sitting with my father trying to match him breath for breath. Maybe we do oamkars for ten or fifteen minutes. He pats me on the back, then disappears into his aqua-colored car. This is the color of the Lebanese family's house down the street. Mr. B. had had paint left over from painting a water tower, so he painted his house aqua. It is terrible to see so much brightness point to another brown family. Why can't the B.'s have a white or beige house? See the brown people, they use leftovers all the time. So I think all the Lebanese are like Indians. Mr. B. using leftover paint on his house reminds me of my father washing and waxing his car. He does not rub all the wax in, feeling that if he can see the wax residue, his car will further benefit from the protection. If he could cover his car with plastic sofa wrap, he would. My father makes me different from white people. This difference is a point of tension in my body.

But every morning, I find myself sitting at his side, inhaling and holding my breath, exhaling and holding my breath, both of us saying "oam"; he in a white T-shirt and shorts, me in orange. I am eight, nine, ten.

There are jars of prescription drugs in our refrigerator. My mother says, "They belong to your father; don't touch."

A memory: We are eating dinner by the map of the world. The phone rings. A patient asks my father for advice. My father says, "Take your painkillers, and I will see you tomorrow."

A dream: My father's dental partner calls my father back to the surgery room to say that one of my father's patients has died under anesthesia. My father had administered this anesthesia. The patient stops breathing. More dreams: My father keeps giving anesthesia to his partner's patients. One dies, then another. They all stop breathing.

Just before my twelfth birthday, my little sister turns five. It is Saturday, and everyone goes to the toy store to buy her presents, while my father stays at home. It is Father's Day. When we return that hot June afternoon, it is so quiet: I can neither go upstairs nor unpack the shopping bags. A few minutes later my brother comes back downstairs and takes my mother upstairs. Then my mother comes back down and instructs all her five children to sit in the basement. We hear sirens and the heavy boots of men thumping upstairs and down.

Is it months later, or only days? I see a newspaper article on the kitchen table. In the first paragraph I see the word *suicide*. This, I think, is a terrible disease like cancer. I don't know if my father left because of suicide of the lungs or bones. My mother uses the word "deseeesed." I wonder why my mother cannot pronounce the word *disease*. For a short while we only go to church. Tight shoes and hard benches. Then we stop going to church. We do not do puja. We do not do oamkar or anything. The precision and suspension of breath I learned from my father, I transfer to counting. I run and count. One-two-three-four. I take up track and cross-country running. I think the morning exercises at the foot of a closet are the ruse of a country no longer near to me. And my father, what does he know, just breathing and disappearing, as if yesterday and tomorrow are the same word, and existence a trick of lighting; *puja, mala,* and *oam* the syllables of my strange name.

4. Asian in the 1970s

The death of my father is for me the beginning of my distrust of yoga. What good is breathing if you just sit in one spot like a dumb lotus, thumbs and forefingers pitched towards emptiness? If I can remember my arrival in America, then I remember disappearing, my dark skin and hair, my black pupils. To affiliate myself with India in the 1970s means I have to negotiate the meaning of being dark in a country that begins with the elimination and containment of one group of darker people and the persecution of another darker-skinned people. To be Indian in a public school in America in the 1970s is to be Native American, what some boys at school call a woo-woo Indian, rain-dance Indian, Indian in a straw hut. To flee from my darkness is to enter the illusion of whiteness, and to enter whiteness is to face something numb, something that can't sing like Aretha, something that tells me to shut off feeling and to keep silent.

For years I reread a book about Martin Luther King Jr. It is a biography written for junior high school children given to my family by Dr. Dan Howard, my father's colleague, and his family. In my mind, I am in love with Martin Luther King Jr. because he is so handsome and smart. Sometimes you get to hear his "I have a dream" speech on the television. Other times the television shows Mr. Nixon and Vietnam, the torn country that is supposed to be mine when I enter the church pews. Then there is King's voice. His voice makes me cry. When I cry, I remember that my father will not be coming home today or tonight. Also, I look at King's picture, and I see the color of my own skin. For a moment I am relieved that I am not ugly. Somewhere along the line, after our arrival in America, it had occurred to me that I was ugly. I learned this from my mother who is very beautiful. I do not have a memory of her telling me whether I was beautiful or ugly. I have a memory of her medicine cabinet. When I open it, there is a pot of cream called Porcelana, something to make her look white. Also, I learn, from my grandparents, that it is not good to linger in the sunshine, sunshine can make you look quite dark and therefore ineligible for the spoils of the world. I am darker than my mother, and my mother is darker than my father. My mother tells me the story of my father's sister-in-law, who says, "Why did Sunder marry a dark girl?" When I look in the mirror I see her face darkened by three days of sunshine.

The more dinner parties my parents have, the more I learn about my father's university. His colleagues are all richer and better dressed than we are. Some of them drive cars more expensive than houses in our neighborhood. Their children go to private schools. When I am in fourth, fifth, sixth grade I want to be as glamorous as Dr. Pinson, Dr. Mohammad, Dr. Howard, and my father's secretary, Mrs. Hezekiah, who is African. All of these people are ten times more glamorous than the white parents in my neighborhood. Also, when I listen to the radio, I hear Diana Ross. It is around this time that I realize to be white is a curious puzzle: You have permission to be average, and you will still succeed, you will get noticed. If you are Asian trying to be white, it goes something like this: You just have to follow along in school and make the grade and be quiet enough so that you don't make any trouble, and nobody will notice that you are a foreigner. In this disappearance, you can start to be white or you can stop being Asian. This is the code of honorary whiteness. To be black is harder. You cannot get away with being average. You have to rise up. You have to be more articulate. You have to have a depth of feeling, your voice comes out with things that sound like the truth. To be Marvin Gaye is harder than to be Donny Osmond. When I see Donny Osmond on the variety shows, I know the world takes no notice of me. When I hear Marvin Gaye, I take notice of myself: I feel that the heavens open up, and we are related. This is strange because just yesterday I remember thinking that Gandhi is Martin Luther King's uncle, the way the older light-skinned guru made way for the younger dark-skinned one. And if this is so, King is my guru, and because he is dead, he is just like my own uncles far away in Bombay, dead. In this space of the dead—which includes King, my country, my languages, my relatives, my father—loss and fantasy dance in my throat, my stomach. This makes breathing very hard for me. Sleeping is also hard. In order to sleep, you have to cry for a long time. When you cry you can remember Marvin Gaye. Also, don't forget Roberta Flack. My mother likes the song "Killing Me Softly." I think this song delivers her back to my father. But that is strange too, because she likes to use bleaching cream on her face, so she can un-Roberta-Flack herself, so she can be porcelain, go out into the street and be eligible for the spoils of the world.

In sixth grade, we are required to submit a poem on the subject of Martin Luther King Jr. I know I will win it because Martin Luther King is my uncle, a part of my breathing. This breathing is happy and sad. The prize is announced, and I win. At the award assembly, held in the cafeteria, I am asked to receive my prize. It is a box of Parcheesi, the "Selchow and Righter Parcheesi, Popular Edition, a Backgammon Game of India." When I walk back to my spot on the floor, I try to cover three words, *Game of India.*

India for me is a limbo between white and black, a limbo of looking in the mirror and seeing what I cannot rub off my skin. It is all the things my father keeps inside a closet; it is the irony of his disciplined breathing—anesthesia, overdose, silence. It is suicide and a foreign language called Hindi, which I do not understand anymore in 1974. It is bright silk clothes, incense, sitar music, and yoga.

For me there are only two choices: Nancy Sinatra and Aretha

Franklin. Aretha Franklin is my first choice. Nancy Sinatra is fine as number two.

It is the 1970s, and yoga belongs to Divali (the festival of lights), to Indian food and soul food, to Kwaanza; belongs to bright clothes on the backs of people the white world punishes then ignores, like people of Vietnam and people of diamond mines. Yoga belongs among buried riches I do not let myself deserve. Two events in America turn me in on myself. The disappearance of my father, and the assassination of Martin Luther King Jr. And it is this sadness that keeps me from anything connected with India, including yoga.

I avoid wearing Indian clothes to school. By the time I am in college I have a vague notion of Divali. I know that the Bhagavad Gita is Krishna's conversation with Arjuna on the nature of duty. It predates *Hamlet* by twenty thousand years, it seems. Krishna is so dark skinned he's blue-black, godly, African. His earthly lover, Radha, is pale, poor, a cow-herding girl, the white-skinned concubine some coiled psyche sent from his paradise. The Kama Sutra is a treatise on lovemaking translated by Victorian men who drink gin neat.

5. The Yoga Sutras

The last months of pregnancy bring me to the slowest form of yoga I have yet practiced. I slow down enough to reenter those first few breathing lessons with my father. I begin to follow along with a less strenuous CD which inspires me to find out more about Patanjali's Yoga Sutras. Dated from around the second century, this is his collection of 195 aphorisms (*sutra* also means "cord" or "thread") which intends to illuminate the essence of yoga (which means "union," "yoke," "vehicle," "method," "aptitude," "trick," "use of equipment"). Patanjali's inspiration comes from the Vedas, and his sutras are recognized by every branch of yoga (hatha, Iyengar, Ashtanga, etc.).

The sutras concern themselves with the causes of suffering and how we can reduce them. The practice of yoga in America focuses on yoga's contribution to physical fitness, in other words the postures or asanas. Interestingly, Patanjali's sutras don't mention any poses. He mentions only the seated posture for meditation. In the fourteenth century, the Hatha Yoga Pradipika lists fifteen mostly cross-legged seated postures. A few hundred years later, a manual called Gheranda Samhita lists thirty-two seated asanas.

My yoga class focuses on standing asanas. I believe that the postures I try to mimic with precise alignment are ancient: two, three, who knows, maybe seven thousand years old. If they are so old, ants, floods, and other weather have destroyed the textual evidence. More likely, these postures are based on modern systems, which in turn base themselves on oral inheritance and an acute concern with the body's energy flows. There is no clear textual lineage. Instead, there are many texts, many more teachers, gurus, yogis, traditions, guides, tastes, and temperaments, many of which may be more recent than we think.

6. The Los Angelization of Yoga

Here is an odd scenario I imagine: Most people who study yoga in America have white teachers.

Here is a fact: Thirty-eight percent of all doctors in America are Indian.

Imagine this: You are East Indian, and you go to your East Indian doctor to help you with your asthma. He prescribes a drug for you. An American pharmaceutical company sells this drug. Your insurance pays for this expensive, long treatment. You go to your white yoga teacher to help you with asthma. She helps design a yoga routine focusing on pranayama and asanas. Your insurance will not pay for this. Ten yoga lessons with this teacher cost 250 dollars.

And yet, learning yoga from white people is, for me, like copying down the ingredients of a vegan lentil dal burger from a Whole Foods deli sticker. I feel there are things I should know, that might have been handed down to me but were not. It is like watching a video on how to drape a sari. It is like seeing so much Indo-chic: hennaed hands on lanky white models in *Vogue,* nose rings, pashmina shawls in *Elle* and on Madonna. I am reminded that in this country there is no father. I inherit nothing. I must acquire my own culture, which includes yours. And you keep acquiring mine.

I replace the yoga classroom with yoga magazines and feel lost in the white media world of exercise and fitness. The Americanization, and more specifically the Los Angelization of yoga seems often to overlook the principal aim of yoga–to eliminate suffering.

The principal aim of a yoga class in L.A.? One can imagine: to flash the visual trappings of health (clear skin, clear eyes, toned muscles, heightened strength and flexibility), to explore alternative body-sculpting methods, to complete, to cruise, to meet, to network, to break into the American quest for rank. To suffer.

The principal aim of L.A. is to mask suffering with the pursuit of illusions. To compete.

Illusion may be a cause of suffering.

The Los Angelization of yoga is not unlike an organic fruit wrapped in twenty thousand layers of nonrecyclable, nonbiodegradable packages, not unlike a sports utility vehicle. We are mobile, we have tasted the pure thing, we have ways to preserve and to run from it. To own it and contain it. To overdo it.

The Americanization of yoga includes strain. A higher rate of injury than from yoga practiced in Asian countries. Emphasis on postures only. Competition. Merchandise: mats, pillows, eye bags, blankets, blocks, ropes, tanks, shorts, T-shirts. J. Crew yoga clothes. Overkill. The terms *power yoga, yoga workout.* Water bottles. Office yoga. Wheelchair yoga. Yoga for athletes. Yoga Web sites. Yoga and body building. Yoga and weight lifting. Yoga becomes something we must own. In our decade, yoga is something to market. To market, to market, the latest way to forget.

Perhaps at the heart of Western thought, particularly American and English thought, is the acquisition and domestication of the material world, and the competitive drive that makes that acquisition possible. In our insatiable drive for ownership and the future, we lose the advantage of the present tense. Thus, we wreck our breathing. Our bodies click out of joint.

The kind of yoga practice which is purely physical is America's lonely encounter with something it does not have the patience or the time to understand. But more than this, it is a lonelier step away from America's own spiritual possibilities. For, by turning at critical junctures to the East–to the stereotype that in Indian philosophy, truth has no social context, that oblivion is the geography of wisdom, that nirvana is emptiness, that nonattachment means we can forget about other people, and about race, class, and gender–America supplies itself with the anesthesia it craves to numb itself from the pain of its history: the pain of stolen land and labor, the outrageous waste. India–like Asia–serves its twisted political function in America. As Richard Rodriguez said, "India beckons." She beckons at certain times. Perhaps as our country begins to enter a plurality, India beckons. In publishing, in fashion, in exercise, we turn not to India, but to "India," the exotic: to Deepak Chopra for example, to the merchandising of yoga. Perhaps this will persist for only a short time. Then someplace else will call America away from its wounds.

This points to capitalism's excess and ignorance, a lack of lucidity about ourselves and about the world. Ignorance is a cause of suffering. Yoga aims to banish ignorance in order to achieve serenity (happiness/peace/compassion). It is a long road. It ought to be traveled without overstraining in the asanas. It ought to be practiced without competitive urges. It ought to be coupled with guidance from a trusted teacher. My teacher is a white woman in Virginia. Over the years, I begin to see a beauty elucidated in the long, fine lines of her body and in her breath and movements. She is an example of the stunning effects of a daily yoga practice that is both physical and linked to the spiritual possibilities that come from cleansing one's body with breath. Somebody like her might have helped my father, who turned to pharmaceuticals, who in the end stopped breathing.

But that is over now. The world, my world, has changed. I inherit the fruits of civil rights, so fierce a struggle in America. It is this movement that makes possible all the diversity in America today. I no longer see my skin in the light of my grandparents' eyes. I no longer associate yoga with the television's backward portrait of India.

7. Poetry and Yoga

As I come to be less apprehensive about the house I am entering, my spine begins to elongate, my fingers spread, my forehead melts in the heat, my hips begin to open. In a few weeks, if I am lucky, I will give birth to my son. I want to pass on to him not the sadness of breathing but the art of it. From Jennifer, from yoga CDs and videos, from Patanjali's Yoga Sutras, I know this: Begin with your breath. You begin where you are. Poetry, like yoga, aims to heighten the awareness of breathing, so that there is space on the page, as between vertebrae, space for the heart and mind to explore and find poise in the unsaid. My father did not come to any conclusion, not in a farewell note, not in his practice of pranayama, not in his career. But I have been given a specific life, the conditions of which are my gift to interpret. From suicide to yoga. From fatherlessness to becoming a mother. I have waited so long to have a child, because I have had trouble breathing, trouble owning my skin. Many things have aided my release. Poetry. Yoga. I have learned to be grateful for the specifics of my life. Pranayama allows my body to be filled with gratitude.

how i became swami mommy
Judith Hanson Lasater

With a last, long, leisurely inhalation and exhalation my morning yoga practice was over. I stretched and got up off my mat to begin my day. This was my routine for years and one which I took deeply for granted. Everyday without fail, I spent more than an hour practicing yoga asana and pranayama. Years of doing this had created a sense of physical well-being. Not only did I benefit from asanas; it was centering in and of itself to have such a consistent routine.

To say everything changed when I became the mother of a

very active baby is an understatement. Not only did I find that a leisurely and predictable yoga practice was now virtually impossible to maintain, but I discovered that any formal yoga practice at all was a challenge to fit into my day.

For a committed practitioner, the need for uninterrupted time each day is a given. But the needs of a young child are varied and unremitting. I think that this is one reason why human beings have traditionally lived in villages with lots of willing hands to help. As a young mother I frequently found myself on the verge of tears; I thought my life would never be about my choices again. I would tell myself that I would forever be at the mercy of a wet diaper and a hungry cry. I felt isolated and yet was afraid that asking for help would be an admission that I did not know how to be a good mother. I struggled for years with this. My goal was to reintegrate spiritual practice into my life the way it had been before I became a mother, but it just wasn't working. I felt stressed when I didn't practice and guilty when I did take practice time "away" from my family. Finally I realized that what I needed to change was not my life but my attitude.

When my first child arrived I was a "yoga teacher who had a child"; over the next few years, as two more children arrived, I became a "mom who taught yoga." I created, which is to say I chose, this shift. I did this out of the understanding that I, in fact, *could* make a shift. I had been prisoner to the idea that my life was being "inflicted" on me. Slowly I came to understand that my life was my own only if I took ownership of it–if I understood my thoughts and feelings as actions rather than reactions. It took me a couple of years to make that shift, but when it happened it was truly transformational. It remains, to this day, one of the most profound asanas I have ever done. My change of attitude allowed me to slowly evolve into someone my kids would later call "Swami Mommy," someone my children would recognize both as their mother and as a committed spiritual practitioner. Here are some of the things I learned along the way.

I learned that my definition of yoga practice was too narrow. In my premommy days, I defined yoga practice very strictly. It was meditation, breathing, postures, and chanting, and nothing more. Now I divide yoga practices into "formal" and "informal." Formal yoga practice is exactly what it sounds like: the specific practices that can be done on the mat or on the meditation cushion. Informal yoga is what happens the rest of the time.

If my only practice time is the couple of hours a day I am meditating or standing on my head, then what happens the other twenty-two hours of the day? In transforming myself into a Swami Mommy I learned that I can take my yoga "off the mat" and into my daily life. Some days I would start a morning headstand, come down out of the pose to fix cereal, and then retire to the living room to resume my headstand, watching while the kids ate. Other days I would lie, hanging half-on and half-off the couch in a supported restorative pose and find myself taking Lego blocks apart while I lay there.

In a more abstract way, I learned that I could "practice" yoga any time I wanted to: The variable was me. I did not need a perfectly clean and quiet room; I could "practice" yoga in the supermarket line, in the car pool, at any time I wanted. If I am a yogini then anything I do is yoga practice. If I choose to remain mindful, then every moment can become a practice.

The first verse of Patanjali's Yoga Sutras, considered by many to be the ultimate source book for the study of yoga philosophy, states: "Atha yoga anushasanam." This translates as "Now the study of yoga (is presented)." This verse has several meanings. It can be interpreted as merely an introduction to the text that will follow. It can also mean that right now, in this very moment, yoga can exist. My practice is not limited by location, but rather by my intention. So this variable can be formed into a question: What am I choosing right now? Am I choosing to practice by remaining aware and mindful, or am I choosing to react with frustration or resentment or disappointment because my yoga practice is not taking the form I would like it to right now? How I answer that question, day after day, shapes my life. When my children were young and things were at their worst, when each of them needed me right now and I felt pulled in three different directions, I would repeat to myself, "It won't always be like this, it won't always be like this." Then I would begin to deal with the

Judith Hanson Lasater

most pressing demand first and somehow the frantic moment would unravel and peace, or something closer to it, would prevail. My focus on mindfulness, even at those times, helped us move into our chosen state of controlled rather than uncontrolled chaos. Another important concept I have learned is that of the sat guru and the upa guru. The term *guru* is made up of the syllables *gu,* which means "darkness," and *ru,* which means "the destroyer of darkness". Thus the guru is one who brings the light of awareness into the darkness of ignorance. Most of us have a mental picture of the classic guru: a kindly older man who suddenly turns and asks the penetrating question that changes your life. But there is also another kind of guru, the upa guru. The word *upa* means "near." The upa guru is whoever is near you at the moment teaching you. And of course that person is teaching you about yourself. Your upa guru may be the person who pulls in front of you in traffic, thus teaching you forgiveness, or the person who helps you pick up your spilled groceries with a smile, thus teaching you generosity, or as it has been so often for me, a child who asks a question or makes a statement that stops me in my spiritual tracks.

Recently I was feeling a bit overwhelmed with the number of things I had planned to accomplish one afternoon, and apparently my stressful demeanor was affecting my environment. My son walked up to me, placed his hands lovingly on my shoulders and said, "Mom, time is big." Instantly I understood his message; time is as spacious as we make it. If I am present in the moment, then I can interpret time to be as "big" as I want. If I interpret time as big, then I can relax the tension in my body and actually learn to enjoy what I am doing. If, on the other hand, I interpret time as small, my body tightens up and I probably will not be able to perform my tasks as well. After all, each moment of my life is potentially as rich as any other if I remain present.

Many times my children have served as upa gurus for me. Another instance occurred when I was remembering some unpleasant experiences from my childhood. My daughter discovered me sitting alone crying. When she asked why and I told her I didn't want to share my suffering with her she said, "But Mom, our feelings are what connect us together. If you do not share your feelings with me, you are keeping us apart." The wisdom of her words was startling. Later, after sharing my experiences with her, I realized that an interaction that had started with me feeling isolated had been transformed into a healing moment. Since that interaction, I have committed to continually trying to see life as a nonstop process of learning. That day I had learned that those we live with and love, even our children, perhaps especially our children, can teach us in a unique way about what it means to be present.

139

Another important lesson I have learned as I have tried to blend the daily spiritual practice of yoga with parenting was that practicing yoga is a blend of abhyasa and vairagyam. *Abhyasa* is the Sanskrit word meaning "disciplined practice"; *vairagyam* means "surrender or detachment." These two concepts are intertwined. It is a little like flying a kite. In order to fly a kite you must do one thing: Let the string out judiciously. If you let the string out too fast (too much vairagyam) the kite crashes. If you do not let the string out at all, the kite cannot fly either (too much abhyasa). Raising kids is like flying a kite: It is about learning when to allow kids to experience and grow from the freedom of making their own mistakes, and when to pull the kite string in and protect them from too much, too soon. Kids need the firmness and consistency of abhyasa combined with the vairagyam of letting go. Wise parenting is the ability to know when to pull in and when to let go. Most of my parenting dilemmas, especially those around raising teenagers, have to do with finding this balance.

This balance is also apparent in practicing a yoga pose. In order to practice it well, some muscles need to let go. But if other muscles do not resist, there will be no stability. It seems to me that we practice to find this balance, and in fact, balance may actually be the practice itself.

Another important thing I have learned about parenting through my yoga practice is that listening is key. When one practices a yoga pose, a dynamic process occurs. First you tell your body what you want it to do. For some students, this is the end.

They then do the pose. But a dynamic practice includes listening to what the body tells you about the effects of the pose. If you listen to your body, you will learn more in the pose. You will learn what to adjust and what to leave alone, where you are tight and where you are just holding on, when the pose is a true physical challenge and when the challenge is mental instead.

Parenting is also about the ability to listen. This listening is more than just receiving sound waves against my eardrums. It is about hearing my child's words with my heart as well as with my ears so that I can hear the feelings and intentions behind the words. If I am sensitive to my body, I can adjust my pose intelligently. If I am sensitive to the feelings that prompt my child's communication I will be able to respond appropriately. Children communicate their needs nonverbally as well. If I focus on their behavior only, and on changing that behavior to meet my needs, I may miss the feelings that are "screaming" behind my child's behavior. If I listen to the feelings I can better understand the needs the behavior is fulfilling. I can then work with my child to help us find new ways of getting his or her need met. When this happens, the behavior will change.

Of course, I am not always able to listen and respond in the way I would like. But I have come to realize that when I can't it isn't about some inherent lack in me or my children. Getting caught up in the moment, being blindly convinced I am right, is intensely human. Yoga has helped by creating a habit of self-reflection. When I "lose it" now I realize it sooner and feel clearer about what I can do to rectify the problem.

One of the startling things I have learned as a parent is that my teenagers need me as much, if not more, than they did when they were young. A similar thing is true of yoga practice. When I was younger, I felt more naturally flexible. I did not feel such a need for stress reduction or relaxation as I do now. As I grow older, my "need" for yoga practice increases. I find flexibility is not such a given; I find I want to spend more time in meditation and less time in anger and distance from the ones I love.

Teenagers may seem very independent, and indeed they are becoming so. But this is the last and crucial stage of parenting. I may not be reading them a good-night story, but I am sometimes called upon for a midnight chat about a personal crisis and the character it takes to do the right thing. In the beginning my yoga practice was more about touching my toes. Now it is about paying attention to what I can learn about myself on the way down there. Parenting is the same. In the beginning it was about changing diapers and protecting my children from falling down the stairs. Later it becomes about letting them try the stairs on their own and changing my attitude as my children become young adults.

The most wonderful thing I have learned about parenting through my years of yoga practice is this: It is not the little aspects of daily practice that matter. In the long run, it is the consistency of practice over years and decades that ultimately shapes my body and mind. So it is with raising children. Consistency over time allows my children the opportunity to feel secure enough to leave me. This will be the proof that I have done my job well. In turn, I hope my practice of yoga will never stop giving me the strength to leave my prejudices and fears and fling myself ever more deeply into life itself. This is what I have learned on my yoga mat and it is what I want to model for my children. It is my gift to them.

journey of a lifetime

Vyaas Houston

श्रेयान् स्वधर्मो विगुणः परधर्मात् स्वनुष्ठितात् ।
स्वधर्मे निधनं श्रेयः परधर्मो भयावहः ॥

Better one's own dharma without merit
Than the other's dharma well executed
Better death in one's own dharma:
The other's dharma is fraught with fear.

—Bhagavad Gita (III.35)

For the two years before I traveled the world with him, I thought of him as a perfect being, a yoga master who was enlightened and all knowing. He was the accomplished Dr. Ramamurti Mishra, a neurosurgeon and acupuncturist, Sanskrit scholar, author, and orator. But for the many years I was with him, he was my guru.

The force that moved me from my life in retreat on Cape Cod to his ashram's gates remains a mystery to me, but from our first meeting it was as if I had entered another realm. I remember arriving for the first time, in the late summer of 1971, at his ashram estate in upstate New York. After walking through an apple orchard and crossing expansive lawns, I noticed a gathering of people. They were seated on the grass, and they faced a small Indian man, who was standing before a blackboard. I stopped at a safe distance, feeling I had come upon something sacred. After a few minutes, I began to feel uncomfortable remaining apart as an observer. As I cautiously approached the back of the group, the teacher stopped the class and asked, "Who is this young man?" My friend, Mary Tasch, who had preceded me, introduced me to Dr. Ramamurti Mishra.

The class resumed and I watched him intently. He was covered from neck to feet in pale orange, which created a striking contrast to the dark color of his hands and face. His handsome features were accentuated by long black hair and his voice was powerfully resonant as he led the group in the chanting of Sanskrit verb conjugations. His presence was electric; he was completely in command.

Later Mary told me that he had given up a lucrative career in medicine to teach yoga psychology and Sanskrit, which he referred to as the science of vibration. Attending the classes and meditations over the next two days I recognized the energy flowing from him to others, and found myself yearning for a look of acceptance. It was not forthcoming. The more I wanted his attention, the more he passed me by. On the second day it finally occurred to me that the only reason I had come here was to learn something. Even as that thought was arising in my mind, he suddenly and immediately shifted his whole attention to me and spoke to me as no one ever had before. I was transfixed.

But I found the philosophical content of Dr. Mishra's talks difficult to understand and I decided to depart for New York City the next day, after the morning meditation. I was packed and ready to leave when he announced that there would be instruction in neti, a yogic nasal cleansing practice. Thinking that this was something I should learn, I decided to postpone my departure a little longer. We entered the kitchen of the main house, and I was shown by one of his assistants how to insert a rubber urinary catheter into one nostril, draw it through the mouth, and move it back and forth while rinsing with saline solution. This was somewhat traumatic, but it was nothing compared with what was to come. After completing both nostrils, I was led into the living room and told to lie down on the floor. Pillows were placed under my shoulders, so my head would tilt back, putting my nostrils in an upright position. Dr. Mishra himself inserted a small vial into each of them. I felt an excruciating fire explode through my sinuses and into my throat. I choked and gagged, and began to writhe, but Dr. Mishra seized my attention by opening my eyes and dropping something into them that created two fine points of such searing pain that I forgot my initial shock. A minute or two later, I sat up. The discomfort of having mustard oil in my nostrils and honey in my eyes began to fade. Still stunned, my vision cleared and I saw Dr. Mishra sitting relaxed in a chair. His penetrating gaze locked in on me, and he asked if I would like to accompany him that afternoon, to Providence, Rhode Island, for a lecture he was giving there. I accepted unhesitatingly.

We set out in two cars. At a rest stop along the way we pulled off, and while I was waiting for the others in the parking lot, I looked up to see Dr. Mishra approaching me. In his hand he carried a black stick about two feet long and an inch in diameter. I realized that I had never seen him without it. The way it fit in his hand as he walked made it seem like an extension of his body, something that added to his mystery. (Later, I discovered that it contained a magnetic steel rod at its core, was covered with black antler bone, and had twenty-five facets symbolizing all the elements of the sankhya yoga cosmology.) As he came closer, I froze. I had no idea how to address this mighty being. But his question to me was simple: "You seem very young man. How old are you?" I told him I was twenty-three, and then to alleviate my discomfort, asked him a question about something he had said in one of his talks. Without answering he turned his back on me. Embarrassed as I was, I instantly understood that my question was not genuine and that Dr. Mishra operated outside the parameters of social conventions.

In Providence I seated myself front and center in the YMCA auditorium. Above me, Dr. Mishra began his program of guided meditation and stories filled with humor and wisdom. As he spoke, I became more and more absorbed, not so much in what he was saying but rather in his presence, which seemed much more dynamic and expanded before this audience of a hundred or so. It was like a journey in which, through him, I experienced a broad range of feelings I had never known before, everything from universal love to the rage of wrathful deities. Throughout his talk I felt as if I were in him and he were in me. When it was over, I was dumbfounded. People gathered for food in the kitchen behind the auditorium but I couldn't consider eating. I didn't know what to do with myself. Dr. Mishra, like a physician matter-of-factly writing a prescription, handed me a glass of warm milk. Drinking it, I knew I had to study with him.

Back at the ashram the next day, I asked for his permission. He told me I was very welcome. Within twenty-four hours I had packed up and said good-bye to my life on the Cape. Upon returning to the ashram I made plans to go to San Francisco, where Dr. Mishra would be teaching at the California Institute of Asian Studies. My excitement was unbounded. I had found a teacher I was sure could lead me to enlightenment. I had also discovered Sanskrit.

I had always been a mediocre student, largely because I could never sustain an abiding interest in any subject. With Sanskrit, I was captivated. I could not get enough. The pure sounds and the intricate symmetry of Sanskrit gave me the feeling that I had come home. It seemed like a universal key that opened my mind and heart to the perfect beauty of life. I had the sense that I would never feel alone and separate again.

In San Francisco, we found a house on sunny Potrero Hill with a large classroom on the ground floor. At the far end of the room was a slightly raised dais, where Dr. Mishra sat behind a small table draped in orange cloth. There, beside his Sanskrit books, he rested his stick as he taught. I picked my spot, five feet to the right and one foot below the place where my teacher sat. There I remained for seven or eight hours a day, every day for the better part of a year, fixated on this man whom, like others in our small group of thirty-odd people, I now called Guruji. Each morning he led us in Kundalini yoga exercises, when through his exhortations to twist and bend further and further to maximum pressure, I would daily discover new extremes of spinal manipulation. He would direct us in his broken English "Hold breath to point of passing out." So I would struggle to hold my breath as long as he did, and it was often very close to the point of passing out. When I did pass out I welcomed it. It released energy that made me "feel every cell pulsating." I learned to feel my blood circulating from "heart to entire body and from entire body to heart." He would refer to the release of chemicals and the release of hidden poisons, and after sustaining a neck twist for a long time, while taking in more and more breath, I would feel an explosion of energy in my brain that made me quiver. Gradually his instructions led to feeling and remaining absorbed in an "ocean of subtle pulsation." He described meditation with the enthusiasm of a sports commentator, sensation by sensation. Yet he described it tenderly, inviting us to embrace our own heart. More than anything he was teaching me how to feel.

Right after meditation we would chant Sanskrit grammar. Following his lead and imitating his sound was something I would never tire of as long as I knew him. His rich resonance vibrated every part of his own body as well as the ocean of pulsation around him. He would bring ancient texts, gods, and sages to life with fluent and brilliant commentary. And he was a great raconteur. When he told a story he inhabited the characters to such an extent that no one could doubt that at that moment he was Krishna, Arjuna, Siva, a goddess, an ancient rishi, or even a terrible asura, enemy of the gods. Many of the stories he told again and again, taking as much delight the hundredth time as the first. His stories were very funny, and no one enjoyed their humor more than Guruji himself. His high-pitched laughter pealed forth, seeming to tickle his every fiber.

Except for a short break, when there was a chance to grab a cup of herbal tea and a handful of sunflower seeds, we went straight through from eight o'clock in the morning until one-thirty in the afternoon, intensively chanting Sanskrit grammar. It pushed me to an edge of discomfort that I thought I couldn't bear for another moment. But I did, every day. When we broke for the one meal of the day I felt tremendous relief. We sat on the floor around a long table, with Guruji at the head. Special tasty dishes had been prepared in small quantities for him and whomever he favored with a spoonful. The rest of us received vegetarian staples prepared by a rotating staff of inexperienced cooks. In the grip of mental exhaustion and physical depletion I found it impossible not to want to sample the guru's delicacies. Moreover, not receiving anything meant rejection and my own inevitable comparison with those on whom he seemed to lavish food and affection. And to make matters still worse, because I craved the food he seldom blessed me. My greed was transparent.

It wasn't just food I wanted. I craved his attention, his approval, and his love. Mostly he withheld it. Only occasionally, when I had given up hope, would he resurrect me with outrageous flattery. That would sustain me for a time, but I longed for more, never considering how much would be enough.

So it went, day in and day out for the next nine months. In spite of my emotional struggles, I was on the fastest learning curve of my life. My belief in Guruji's unflawed mastery only increased. I never saw him miss a beat, lose his concentration, or be at a loss for words in any situation. He was tireless, teaching seven days a week, five hours in the morning and another two and half, sometimes three or four, in the evening. I believed he was working overtime for one purpose: our, my, enlightenment.

In the summer of 1972, all my hard work in Sanskrit reached a point of maturation. For the first time, I was translating independently. To my joy and amazement, I also found that I had won myself a place in Dr. Mishra's inner circle. In September Guruji gave me a difficult translation to work on. It was a challenging next step for my Sanskrit, and it was perfectly timed. For the better part of the next year I worked devotedly on a translation of the *Siva-Mahimnah Stotram*, an ancient collection of verses that poetically describe the mythology of Siva. Guriji asked me to tran-

scribe and edit his commentary from lectures, which both interpreted the stories of Siva and elaborated on many of his own. At
about the same time, Guruji began to divide his time between
teaching Sanskrit and acupuncture. Although I recognized his
gift as a doctor I was not inspired to study acupuncture in the
same way as Sanskrit. In my attempts to be a loyal disciple, I initially attended the classes, but found it difficult to concentrate,
and eventually found reasons not to be there. As I watched my
friend Mary work towards her acupuncture license, I had some
doubts about my loyalty, but by that time I had begun to differen-
tiate myself as an individual, distinct from Guruji, with my own
interests and pursuits.

In the fall of the following year we found out that Guruji
would be taking a world tour by ship. Mary and her husband
Fred were concerned about his traveling alone and recom-
mended to Guruji that I go along on the trip for support. When he
agreed to the need for a companion I was ecstatic. After two
years of devoted service, I was chosen to accompany him, support him, carry his luggage, and attend to his needs. I believed
that this would be the greatest blessing of my life.

In mid-January of 1974, we departed by ship from Fort Lauder-
dale. The ship was a radical departure from my familiar ashram
life. I was an obvious disciple, dressed all in white, following my
orange-clad Indian guru around the decks of the ship, and I felt
conspicuous. But aside from the considerable amount of time
spent eating, I saw little of Guruji, who remained in his cabin
much of the time. I managed to pass some time by working on a
translation of the Bhagavad Gita and watching the giant swells of
the ocean, but away from the routine of daily classes and group
dynamics, I was bored and lonely. Guruji suggested that I offer a
yoga class, so I spoke to the activities director, and she scheduled
it in the ship's bar for the next afternoon. More than a hundred
people showed up, and I managed to teach a successful class.
When I saw Guruji later at dinner, I told him, "You taught a good
class today." It fell flat. There was no agreement on his part. I had
come up with this statement, because of the idea propagated in
the culture of yoga and, I believed, by Guruji himself, that the

guru works through the disciple. But it also exposed my ongoing effort to have him think highly of me, a project doomed to failure, not because he didn't, but because of his refusal to participate in stroking my ego.

During our first week at sea, I tried to be useful and offered to wash and iron Guruji's clothes. Although it was tedious work, I took satisfaction while pressing his orange kurtas and lunghis from being a good disciple, engaged in selfless service to my teacher. But after I had twice returned a neat pile of pressed garments, he informed me he'd be doing his own laundry from now on. I was sure he had picked up on both my motive and my resistance.

We arrived in Southampton after a week at sea, and spent two dreary days in London. When we reboarded, Guruji had been assigned a new cabin with a porthole in the rear of the ship. As soon as we left port, we hit a terrible storm. Since Guruji and I had already gotten our sea legs, we were practically the only passengers appearing for meals in the dining room. All around us unsecured plates were flying off tables and shattering on the deck. The first night of the storm I awoke in the middle of the night perspiring and trembling with fear. The ship's roll had become almost vertical as it slid down the face of gigantic waves. Concerned about Guruji, I threw on some clothes and made my way through empty corridors to his cabin. I knocked and called his name, and after some time he opened the door. His response, although polite, made me feel that my call was an unnecessary interruption.

The next day he began to dictate a letter describing the strange experience he had been having since the beginning of the storm. Staring out his porthole, seeing the red color of sunset on the horizon, he had envisioned all humanity burning in the fires of human suffering. As he spoke he seemed greatly changed and moved by the experience. It was as if the vision persisted within a more expanded inner space of his being. Connecting to this oceanic depth of feeling in him as I wrote down his words, I felt reverence, and peace.

Each time we stopped in port, I would carry for him a shoulder bag that weighed at least twenty pounds. At first I was honored to perform this service, but with time as I became familiar with its contents, namely all the official documents and diplomas he had accumulated in a lifetime, I began to regard the lugging of this heavy bag everywhere we went as totally unnecessary. My doubts about his perfection had begun to form. Although I never said a word, he clearly sensed my resistance, and began to carry the bag himself.

When we landed in a port, after a week or two at sea, we would have a full day ashore. I discovered that Dr. Mishra did not believe in queues, and would cut in front of hundreds of people, waiting in line to disembark. Pretending to be invisible, I followed his lead, justifying it as a special guru privilege. I also learned that his personal preference for sightseeing was to get on a local bus, take it to the end of the line and back, then catch a different bus and repeat the same. All the while, we seldom talked. In fact, he asked me to sit apart from him. To me it was painfully boring. By the time we reached our final port in Auckland, I was relieved to have completed this part of the journey. Discontent had set in as doubts continued to surface about my traveling companion. Relieved of my duties and unable to communicate with anyone as a peer amounted to an identity crisis for me. What exactly was my role to be?

Two events that occurred in Auckland set the tone for the next couple months of travel. The first concerned Guruji's considerable luggage, including seventy pounds of books; the second a cheese sandwich.

The ship had had unlimited portage. For the next leg of the journey, however, we would be traveling by air. Anything over forty pounds would be heavily surcharged. Moreover, I would have to the carry the extra baggage. I urged him to ship the books back to San Francisco and we checked the rates at a local shipping office. It seemed settled. That afternoon we visited the Auckland zoo, where Dr. Mishra decided to have some lunch. He ordered the only vegetarian item on the snack bar menu, American processed cheese on white bread, which I regarded as inedible. I found this intolerable. He couldn't wait to eat until we found a decent restaurant. In protest I sat with him at the outdoor table refusing to eat. Then, when we returned to the hotel, Guruji informed me that he would be taking the books on to Fiji with him. I became enraged and stormed out of the hotel. For hours I wandered the streets of Auckland, brooding over these events. I couldn't accept that my teacher was so attached to his books or that I would have to carry them. I went over it again and again in my mind, unable to resolve my frustration. When I returned to the hotel, I found that Guruji himself had taken all his bags to the airport freight office, and had them shipped ahead to Fiji. Imagining his struggle with the huge bags, I felt remorse for my pettiness and failure to be there to help him.

On route to Fiji, my shaming was complete, when he informed me that he had wanted to give the books away to people we would meet there. We later discovered that Guruji's books had been lost. I thought at the time that my anger was responsible for the disappearance of the books. I think he thought so, too.

Our trip was becoming a journey of disillusionment. The Dr. Mishra that I traveled with was very different from the great teacher I had known before, and I was having anything but the trip of a lifetime I had imagined. Since our journey began, I had only become more and more aware of his deficiencies. But in Fiji he had a large audience of Indian people, starved for spiritual nourishment from their mother India, and he shone once again in all his glory. Speaking in his native Hindi, he became completely free in his expression. His talks literally sang. His speech was musical and rhythmic, rising and falling with great waves of energy. He was in his element—far more so than when teaching Westerners.

When he wasn't lecturing, he treated anyone who came to him with acupuncture. Our little cottage on the bay behind Suva's Grand Hotel became a clinic, where people lined up for relief from their diabetes and heart problems. In a short two weeks, he became a hero to the people there. I remember a doctor there, a distinguished-looking man, saying, "We have a very learned man in our midst." Inspired by what I saw, I told Guruji that I thought I should study acupuncture.

"See," he replied. "We have to follow our destiny."

I instantly abandoned the idea.

We continued our journey, to Singapore and then the Philippines. There we traveled to a luxurious mountain retreat in order to meet the famous psychic surgeon Dr. Tony Agpaua. When we were granted an audience with him nothing of note occurred. Dr. Mishra tried to make conversation, but got little response. Quickly, it was over, except that Guriji wanted to have his picture taken with Dr. Tony. By that time we had been traveling for more than two months and he knew I had not brought a camera. But he became furious when I was not able to take this picture. Why, he asked me angrily, had I come with no camera? To spare us all the embarrassment, a kind man offered to take the picture and send us a copy. Everyone stepped outdoors in the sunlight, and the two doctors posed uncomfortably together while the snap was taken.

Our next stop was the capital city of Taiwan, Taipei. For a week Guriji studied at an acupuncture clinic, while I rested a knee injury, caused during a yoga demonstration at a school in Fiji. He seemed annoyed that I wasn't sightseeing. I was annoyed that he didn't just give me some acupuncture. Finally he took me to the free clinic. In a crowded room of about fifty practitioners, a student administered four prescribed needles, as Guruji looked on. As he turned the last needle, I felt a circuit of electricity move around my knee. When I got up, I knew the knee had been cured. I was amazed, and wondered if Guruji had anything to do with it. Though my mistrust of him continued to grow, I did not doubt his gifts.

We moved on to Hong Kong, where Guruji purchased large quantities of acupuncture supplies. When we arrived in Bangkok, we discovered that the bag containing the equipment had not arrived. On further inquiry, we realized that the bag had never been checked in. It had been stolen while we were waiting in line at the Hong Kong airport. Guruji was more upset than I had ever seen him. He could not help blaming me, questioning why I had come if not to make sure all bags were properly checked. It was true; I had forgotten the original purpose of my coming. Our relationship had changed so much. I felt very badly about his considerable loss, but couldn't accept full responsibility for it. To make matters worse, Guruji had left his black stick in the airport. It was the first time in nearly three years that I saw him without his stick in hand. We immediately took a taxi to the airport, but the stick was not to be found. Nothing could have brought home to me more the extent of his turmoil over the original loss than for him to lose his stick. Without it he seemed exposed, like a wizard unprotected by his wand.

After a short stopover in sleepy Rangoon, the capital of Burma, we flew across the Bay of Bengal and landed in Calcutta. It was late April, the beginning of the hot season. I was awed by what I saw: vast numbers of people everywhere, all seeming to move and breathe together in one continuous field of life. There was no way for me define what I was seeing and feeling. I had left the world as I knew it, with its orderly sense of time and space. Guruji, in the mood to celebrate our arrival, asked me if I would like to try some liquid marijuana. It had been five years since I had tried any kind of intoxicant; they had all dropped away when I had dedicated myself to yoga. But now I felt eager to try something that would break up the weary monotony of constant travel. We went to a shop operated by the Indian government, and there drank a tall glass of a strong but pleasant-tasting greenish liquid, known as bhang. We then set out for Dakshineshvara, a temple on the banks of the Ganga, which in the nineteenth century had been the home of the great mystic Ramakrishna. It was after visiting the temple that I began to feel the effects of the bhang. We were driving along the banks of the Ganga, and the heat was stifling. Dust from the road began to pour in through the windows. Guruji was waxing poetic about the sacred Ganga, flowing from the locks of Lord Siva, high in the Himalayas. I began to feel very disoriented, overwhelmed by the intensity of India. What was I doing here, I wondered, and who was the strange man seated to my left? Then I noticed that I was very dehydrated. My mouth was parched. I rolled up the window, shutting out the dust. The heat became claustrophobic. I rolled it down.

When we got to the airport I headed directly to the nearest

water station. We took our bags to a bench in the center of the grand lobby of the airport. Guruji, intent on leaving for New Delhi that evening, told me to stay with the luggage while he checked our tickets. As I sat, the bhang began to feel stronger than I could bear. The water had done little to hydrate me. I was desperate for more water but afraid to leave my location, for fear of getting lost. It was as if I were seeing the vast airport teeming with people through the eyes of a small child. I felt lost, alone, and barely able to hang on. After what seemed an interminable time, Guruji returned with the tickets and sat down to my left. After a minute or two he turned to me and asked me if I was all right. Not wanting to concern him, knowing his resistance to spending a single night in Calcutta, I decided I would manage by following his lead. I told him I was. But my discomfort only increased. Another few minutes passed. He turned to me again and asked if I were sure I was all right. I told him the truth. I didn't see how I could possibly fly that night.

After changing the tickets Guruji told me to pick up my bags and follow him. Somehow I managed to do this. We entered an office with a man sitting at a large desk. A register was before him. At least eight other men were standing around the office leaning against the walls. Guruji sat on the other side of the desk. I was given the other chair next to the registrar. Immediately I asked if I could please have some water. Then the discussion began. Guruji was trying to procure two single rooms in the government hotel. Examining his book, the registrar said that only a double was available. Sitting across the desk from him, I watched Guruji's face as he negotiated. I knew he had taken an even stronger dose of bhang than I, and yet here he was, a master of every facial muscle, oozing charm with a smile that could melt anyone's resistance. It was like watching a great actor on the big screen. Momentarily I forgot my suffering. I was amazed that the registrar did not submit immediately. He continued to insist that a double was the only thing available. Then Guruji dramatically concluded his argument by pointing at me.

"Will you just look at this boy? Do you think anyone can spend the night with someone in his condition?"

I felt a penetrating examination of me by all the eyes in the room. The registrar looked back to Guruji and asked, "What is his condition?"

Guruji's reply shocked me. "You see, he is a devotee of God. Today, he visited Dakshineshvara, the place of Paramahansa Ramakrishna, and there he went into state of divine intoxication. No one can be with him while he is like this."

It hit me like the monsoon after a year of drought. It was the funniest thing I had ever heard in my life. I rocked back and forth with laughter. The last thing I remember was someone handing me a glass of water.

155

Soon we were driving out into the country and arriving at a small hotel. I was shown to my private room. Wooden shutters were opened. Into the room flowed the soft light of the setting sun, the sweet sounds of birds and crickets and a gurgling stream, from which arose the cool fragrant air of evening. My first day in India ended in profound peace. Gratitude filled my heart.

The feeling continued the next morning as we rode in a rickshaw at dawn over the ancient land. Rarely had I experienced such beauty and tranquillity. That afternoon we arrived in New Delhi and took a bus directly to Haridvar, where India's greatest festival, the Kumbha Mela, had just taken place at the location where the holy river Ganga first meets the plains. For the first time I saw naked sadhus, covered in ash and carrying tridents like their beloved Siva, marching down the center of the street. It was so strange that there seemed to be only a thin line between waking and dreaming. The next morning we wandered through a labyrinth of alleyways that formed the extensive bazaar of Haridvar. Shopkeepers were still rolling up the corrugated doors of their garage stalls, elevated two steps above the narrow street. There were entire shops filled only with conch shells, or religious statuary, incense, and marigold garlands around candles in leaf boats to be offered to the Ganga. As we continued our tour of the bazaar, the late-morning Indian sun overwhelmed me. I needed water. Guruji told me there was one more shop to visit. I watched him go up the steps of a stall, and still standing on the street, I was amazed when I looked up to see hundreds of canes covering its walls, many of which were made of the exact same black antelope horn as Guruji's. Before I could collect myself from the shock, Guruji was holding out to me three sticks identical in every detail to his own.

"Which one?" he asked. The thought raced through my mind, How can he be asking me? How could I possibly know? But in the meantime I had become entranced by the three sticks he held forth in his open palms. The one in the middle definitely stood out, with a strength and luster the others lacked. Without hesitating I pointed to it. "That one." He took hold of it and waved it in the air while I savored the glimpse that he had given me of my power to choose.

That afternoon, we departed for nearby Rishikesh in the Himalayan foothills, the final hill station on the Ganga before its waters reached the plains. Here we set up a base for the two months we planned to stay in India. Guruji returned to stay at a dharmashala he had visited often as a child, accompanying his mother. Wanting solitude, Guruji had arranged for me to stay at an ashram a mile upstream. Each morning I would return to his rooftop abode to find him facing a window open to the Ganga, absorbed in meditation. I always noticed that his room, wherever it happened to be, had an atmosphere of purity and clarity. Walking into it, I felt uplifted, as though a new day was beginning afresh.

Daily we went on long excursions. Often at midday, when other sensible Indians had sought shade from the unrelenting heat, we would be riding along in a rickshaw, or climbing the long steps to a temple, or wandering through the marketplace. I had long since tired of following Guruji about. Our unresolved tensions were now compounded by the unparalleled hardships of travel in India in the hot season. His impatience with me matched my irritation with him. I thought more and more of leaving him, venturing off into the Himalayas. I began to read articles by J. Krishnamurti that drove home the individual's need to reject all forms of authority, especially gurus, if one was ever to know freedom. When other students arrived from the states, I vented my frustrations. But the more I thought about leaving him, the more I realized what a hold he had over me. Although I broke away for a few days at a time to escape the heat by going to higher altitudes, I could not bring myself to simply leave him.

One day it all changed. At mid-morning I arrived at Guruji's cottage, to find him curled up on his side, his knees pulled into his chest, obviously not feeling well. All the love and respect I had had for him before we began our travels came flooding back, and my only desire was to help him. I set about cleaning his rooms and washing his floors. I decided the best remedy would be a wholesome meal of dal, rice, and vegetables. I found what I needed in the marketplace, including some mild digestive spices. Some doubts arose when I entered the tiny primitive kitchen on the roof of the dharmashala, but somehow I managed to get the coal stove going and prepare the meal. It was the first really nourishing home-cooked meal we had had in a long time. When I left at the end of the day Guruji was feeling better and the tension that had built between us dissolved. But more than that, cleaning, shopping, and cooking for him turned out to be the act of love that freed me.

The next day when I returned, I found the roof busy with activity. Members of his family had arrived from their village, including his elder sister, his wife, and his nephew. Surrounded by them Guruji seemed more relaxed and content than I had ever seen him. And on that day, for the first time, there was a natural ease between us that would last for the duration of our stay in India. When we traveled again together to Delhi and Bombay, it was as friends. For that short time of our long journey together we shared a feeling of oneness.

I decided to stay on in India, while Guruji kept his plan to return to New York in late June. Shortly before he left, his son Omkar came to be with him. Aside from the age difference of about forty years, they were identical in feature. Everywhere we went, Omkar dutifully carried his father's heavy bag. Sitting across from them at an outdoor cafe in Delhi, I watched Omkar as he stared at his father. His love held nothing back. It wanted nothing, except, of course, his father's love.

The journey held all the pieces of our long relationship, the lessons I would repeat again and again. When I tried to follow his path, mine became conflicted. When I deified him, I became afraid of his power and critical of his imperfections. Yet he saw in me possibilities that no one else seemed to perceive. In many ways he honored me, and changed the course of my life. When I looked at him as a human being, I saw he was quite fallible. But only upon seeing that could I say that I truly loved him. Simple friendship did not come easily with Dr. Mishra, but when we met from time to time in later years, we felt joy upon seeing each other.

the guru question

Jeff Martens

Long ago a farmer in desperate need of water for his crops started digging a well into the hard earth. When he had dug the hole deep enough to cover his head without success, the farmer climbed out of the hole and started to dig another. Soon the days turned into weeks. Six-foot holes began to dot his property. Still, the farmer kept digging new holes until, tired and exasperated, he would toss his shovel aside at the end of each day, climb out of the hole and walk home with the setting sun. Each night he would fall into bed with the scent of damp earth in his nostrils and dream the promise of clear, cool water before waking to dig a new hole the following morning.

One day a neighbor made a rare visit to the farmer's land, his brow raised at the site of so many holes.

"What on earth are you doing?" the neighbor called down to the farmer.

"I'm digging a well," the farmer replied.

"But you will never find water that way!"

"What do you mean?" asked the farmer. "To find water, I have to dig a well!"

"That may be so," answered the neighbor. "But the water table here starts ten feet below the surface. Unless you dig deeper you'll never find what you're looking for."

The essence of this tale has repeated itself many times in my head. When I first heard this story several years ago I had a strong vinyassa practice and was teaching nine yoga classes per week. I felt that I had come to a plateau with my asana and meditation practice and was once again digging for a new way to expand my experience of vivekakhyati, or true discernment. Hearing the story of the farmer and his many wells bothered me at first in a way that I couldn't quite figure out. As it was told to me, the story was meant to signify the importance of sticking to one teacher or spiritual path rather than sampling many different paths or gurus in a shallow manner. If you don't persevere with one guru, the story goes, you will never go deep enough to reap any true benefits. Taking in the story's meaning was a mildly unpleasant experience for me, a bit like swallowing a grain of sand. Almost immediately I found myself tapping into that familiar vein of doubt which I had come to know as my "Guru Question." I wondered once again about the need for a personal teacher or guru in my daily life.

At times I have felt a strange sort of envy for those yogis and spiritual seekers who could refer to their teacher with impunity as a lifelong guru. Usually these individuals would start their sentences with, "Well, *my* teacher says . . ." and proceed to demonstrate a sureness that seemed beyond question. It wasn't as if I had never studied with significant yoga teachers in my own life. Indeed it has been my good fortune to study with many great teachers in several spiritual disciplines, all of them linked together like pearls on the single strand of yoga or divine unity. My inner appetite for mystical Christianity, Taoism, Kabbalah, and Buddhism had allowed my spirit to blossom with full and heartfelt realizations. Yet so often in my life I had come to a point, whether it was after a few months or several years, when I felt it necessary to make a break from my teachers in order to find my own way.

The story of the farmer and his many wells forced me to look at this practice of striking out on my own in a way that raised new doubts. By not embracing and sticking with one particular guru, was I becoming like the farmer digging his many wells? Was my search for enlightenment only creating more darkness? Are we not all born with our own personal connection to divine guidance? Was my search for vivekakhyati doomed to failure without the guidance of my own personal living guru? At the time I heard about the farmer's wells, the issues raised by these questions functioned as the cornerstones of my existence. The more I took them out to study for possible answers, the more the foundation of my current beliefs began to tremble. Soon I became so caught up in examining these questions that I neglected to notice how much the structure of my beliefs was swaying and how close I was coming to a radical fall.

While studying Patanjali's Yoga Sutras for an answer to my Guru Question, I was reminded that ignorance or suffering occurs when the mind mistakes transient perceptions of the outside world for ultimate reality. In other words, our senses reveal a world that we expect to see based on past experience rather than the way the world actually is. According to Patanjali, this is known as avidya or "incorrect comprehension." Avidya is the inherent result of seeking our true identity and worthiness exclusively in the outside world. Caught in the web of avidya, we mistakenly assume that we will be at peace if we can only get all the outside details of our lives to be just right.

The problem with this approach is that the outside world rarely, if ever, conforms to the expectations of our ego. When one person or situation "fails" to meet our expectations, we constantly look in a new and different direction that only appears new and different. In reality, our choices are made through the preset limitations of past experience. Our present actions are then reduced to mere reactions through raga, excessive attachment, and dvesa, excessive aversion. As a child, for example, I suffered severe bouts of chronic illness. Born with a total lack of gamma globulin A, I was doomed by the medical profession to live a life filled with asthma, antibiotics, and upper respiratory infections. As an adult these infections manifested themselves deep in my sinuses. A simple cold would turn into months of exhaustion and intensive antibiotic treatment. Yearning to be free and healthy, my dream was to get sick and then get better quickly like a "normal person" would.

In the state of avidya, our lives become a circular path chasing one thing while avoiding another. Original thought and action are nearly obliterated as we crave repetition to avoid unexpected or unfamiliar sorrows. Without truly breaking any new ground inside where it counts, we frantically dig many holes of distracting experience in the outside world, hoping that this time we will find that peace and sense of wholeness and fulfillment we so desperately seek. On this wheel of samskara or illusion, chasing after pleasure only brings us more pain.

We are bound to the wheel of incorrect comprehension by our attachments and repulsions. For many years my attachment to my illness was as powerful as my yearning to be well. Since I experienced all my thoughts and interactions through the familiar filter of my own dis-ease, part of me held on to illness as a familiar way of living my life with no surprises. The state of constant illness had become my way of relating to the outside world. It was familiar and therefore oddly comfortable. Having a chronic illness forced me to push harder in order to appear to be as "normal" as everyone else. This pushing only led to more and more prolonged states of dis-ease. Going to a job and pursuing a degree in a field I didn't like, not listening to my body, ignoring my emotions, and a secret, growing self-pity led me deeper and deeper into the spiral of illusion, which strengthened my incorrect comprehension about myself and the world around me. I had yet to learn that safety does not have to equal the familiarity of digging yet another unsuccessful six-foot well.

Yoga teaches us that the way to counter the state of samskara is to enter a state of divine contemplation on the nature of our true identity. Known as dhyana or meditation, this practice requires the development of one-pointed concentration, known as dharana. By sticking with the path of letting go of one's own self-importance, one achieves samadhi, blissful absorption with the object of contemplation. Once this is accomplished, beauty is truly in the eye of the beholder, since we create beauty and grace and love by our very gaze. As the Zen saying goes, once you are enlightened, the whole world becomes enlightened. In a state of samadhi, we see our own inner perfection reflected by the entire world. Yet this task, according to many teachers and spiritual texts, requires such a drastic shift in awareness that a living guru or mentor is needed to guide us through the minefield of our own doubt. It seems that the guru's role is much like that of training wheels when we first learn to ride a bike. Their mere presence helps to supplant all doubt as they show us what is possible. They incubate our divine identity for us until we develop the faith and strength and knowingness to claim that divine realization of unity within ourselves.

Choosing one path or guru and sticking with it, the farmer's story tells us, is the only way to dissolve the transient world of illusion in order to rediscover our true source and destination. Soon my struggle against this answer started to affect my yoga practice in subtle ways. A forgetful moment here, a stepping out of the posture there. Instead of experiencing present-moment awareness, my mind began to indulge in samsaya, doubt, about my teaching, my practice, and my life. The story I had swallowed like a light grain of sand now rested heavily, pulling at the very root of my awareness. At the core of the farmer's story I found a direct passageway to my own spiritual journey in search of the ultimate guru, my own vast field of six-foot wells which I had been digging as long as I could remember.

Asking questions without becoming silent to hear the answer is the perfect fertilizer for fear and doubt. New questions sprouted from my dark field of doubt like weeds in light of the farmer's story. Was this not the New Age, the Age of Aquarius? Was I not now living in the Western world? Was not the time for seeking enlightenment by sitting in a cave alone now coming to a close in favor of a new time of group consciousness, in which we serve others by letting our own inner light shine? Was latching onto a guru as a substitute for my higher self the only way to realize the divine nature of my own existence? And then came the familiar topper for me that always plunged me into a state of true frustration. Was not the entire world an expression of ultimate reality (satyada) as much as it is an expression of samskara or illusion?

By this time the story of the farmer was pulling at my yoga practice to the point of complete distraction. Wrapped in layer upon layer of questions, the slight grain of awareness that I had originally swallowed from the farmer's story was now challenging my worldview from the inside out. Already questioning the ultimate purpose of asana, I now found myself doubting the very foundations of a yoga practice. How would doing a better triangle or headstand bring me to enlightenment? What was the purpose of all this asana anyway? Feeling disillusioned with my belief system in the validity of multiple gurus seriously threatened, my questioning of the story's premise took on an even more defensive tone. Had I not already had many gurus? Was not the world my guru? Every flower? Every formal teacher? Every so-called enemy?

For the first time in my life I began to truly doubt the validity of yoga as a path to freedom. My mind set to work to maintain my concepts of the world and my spiritual path so that I could once again return to my familiar grasp of reality. My constant seeking for an answer led me to the decision that I would restructure the story of the well. This new version of the well story was to become my personal touchstone. At the time I considered it to be the ultimate summation of my yoga practice.

My revision of the story went something like this: I was the farmer digging the well. But rather than many different holes, each teacher or spiritual path I had experienced represented a different digging tool rather than a different hole. This practice allowed me to dig deeper and deeper, concentrating on one hole all along. In this model, my study of Kabbalah and the mystery schools of Christianity became a pitchfork and a shovel. My study and practice of yoga became a pick. My meditations on the Dhammapada, the Upanishads, and the Bhagavad Gita all became different implements for digging deeper into the mystery of my being, as did the myriad of formal teachers and disciplines that had come into my life. The hole I was digging became my self, my true self. My surrender and devotion was to the path of vivekakhyati, true discernment, rather than to one particular guru or teaching.

After months of internal struggle, this new version of the story allowed me to make a temporary peace with myself. I could now view the well story as a diverse path of nonconformity without emphasizing attachment to any one particular guru. For a while, a brief while, I sat back with an air of self-contentment, believing that I had found "the answer." But though I was able to reengage my familiar way of viewing and interacting with the world, something felt very different, as if I was trying to squeeze into old clothes that no longer fit me.

Finding an "answer" on the spiritual path is a tricky thing. By answering something we often attempt to stop the wheel of samsara long enough for the outside world to conform to our idea of how we think the world should be. My first clue that I hadn't found true peace with this subject came with a new wave of doubt the next time I taught an asana class. All around me students were moving their bodies in challenging ways, and I found myself viewing them through what could only be described as a filter of despair. What was the purpose of all this asana anyway? I asked myself, and had to literally pause to refocus in the middle of class.

Though I felt myself standing once again on the familiar ground of past belief, the old foundation of my spiritual journey now felt hollow and fragile, as if it were about to crumble away under the slightest inspection. When the Guru Question rose to the surface again I responded by ignoring it and plunging deeper into my asana practice. I looked at myself in the mirror less. Balancing postures became more difficult. I had to struggle mightily to maintain dharana, one-pointed concentration.

One danger of engaging in the practice of yoga is that we can become conditioned to our practice. The possibility exists that we will expect our practice to be a certain way and provide us with certain results. I had met several teachers and students over the years who seemed to be dependent and almost addicted to their practice, going so far as to claim that they couldn't live without their weekend fix of asana. When practiced without present-moment awareness, asana can become just another stop on the wheel of pleasure and pain. How, I wondered, would my asana practice ever lead me to an enlightened state, if what I was doing was creating more expectations, addictions, and aversions? Was I using my practice to dig yet another six-foot hole? Would having my own guru lead me out of this predicament? Or would it just take me further into someone else's form and practice, which I would merely adopt as my own?

Though I was normally adept at asanas, my physical practice began to suffer. I lost tapas, or passion and dedication to my path. Taking my proficiency of asana for granted, I practiced the physical postures less and less and became caught up in the demands and struggles of the outside world. Teaching yoga at the university level and organizing an international yoga conference became a poor substitute for asana and pranayama. In the end, my revision of the farmer's story had only produced deeper questioning. Exploring the role and place of the guru in the modern Western world became my personal crusade to defend the absence of a traditional guru in my own life. My meditation sessions became intellectual wrestling matches with the lack of a formal guru. Snared deep in the web of avidya, I slowly began to give up my meditation and asana practice with the idea of giving my body and mind a break.

As Krishna tells Arjuna in the Bhagavad Gita, quitting is not an option. Giving up my yoga practice only increased my sense of inner turmoil. Somewhere inside I continued to rebel mightily at the idea that just sticking with one guru was the only answer. The process of taking in this bit of wisdom felt as if I had swallowed a rock. Indigestible and lacking any apparent nutritional value, the blatant meaning behind the story of the six-foot wells sat at my navel point and simply refused all my attempts to reason, analyze, or justify it away. I could hardly guess at the time that the mind-based pursuit of my Guru Question would lead me to a most profound experience, a boulder-sized pearl of realization that would reconnect me to my yoga practice in a way I could never have imagined. Most unexpected of all, it was a deep physical experience, a learning on the cellular level and not a sudden mental understanding, which led me to a new frontier of peace, a state more real than any level of intellectual analysis could ever hope to attain. When clarity finally struck on this cellular level, it came with such an impact that it literally took my breath away.

Early one winter morning after struggling with my Guru Question for many months I found myself outside doing some yard work. At this point I had all but abandoned my morning asana and meditation practices. Working outside gave me some degree of peace, allowing me to focus on something else besides the constant churning of my own mind. Perhaps as a symbolic gesture, I felt compelled to clear away clutter and get rid of everything that my wife and I didn't need. Opening a storage shed, I saw a large, heavy roll of old carpet which needed to be thrown out. Grabbing the end of the roll, I started to drag it across the backyard, lifting as much as I could to make the process easier. Almost immediately I felt a gentle tug in my right groin. As I continued to pull the carpet toward the gate, a memory surfaced clear as the morning sun.

When I was sixteen I had a job working at a catalog showroom. A woman came into the store and bought a heavy weight set that came in one large box. I remembered wheeling the weights out to her car in a cart. I remembered reaching into the cart and lifting out the box, determined to do this on my own. I remembered feeling something give in my right groin. With a mighty heave I placed the weights into her trunk. I walked back into the store sensing an odd looseness inside my lower right abdomen. A week later I was in a doctor's office. Groin strain was the diagnosis. Rest and asking for help with heavy lifting was the cure.

As I finished pulling the carpet into the front yard, the tug in my right groin turned into a persistent twinge. At last I set the carpet down at the curb and felt the area above the right side of my pubic bone. I was surprised to feel a golf-ball-sized bulge in the area of the inguinal canal. A sensation of pressure began to swell beneath the skin. Walking back into the house I passed my wife Michele, a massage therapist who was busy answering e-mails at the computer. I moved quickly into the bedroom, thankful that she was too busy to notice my concern. Lying on the floor, I became conscious of my psoas and decided to do some restorative postures. I never made it past the first cycle of Pavan-muktasana.

The twinge in my groin quickly bloomed into a throbbing sensation that shot through my sacrum. The pain was now strong enough to affect my breathing. Michele entered, saw my state, and slowly helped me onto the bed and a heating pad. With her touch and calming words I felt the first wave of pain subside. I assured her I would be all right and told her it was okay to go back to the computer. My experience of healing myself of my chronic infections had taught me beyond a doubt that our thoughts create our physical experience. Working to catch my breath, I started to focus on a process of deep relaxation.

There is something very honest about intense physical pain. Its urgency helps clear away the mental clutter of all that is not essential and throws you deep into the present moment. In a matter of just a few breaths the abnormal bulge above my right groin swelled to the size and consistency of a billiard ball. The level of pain was fast approaching what only moments before had seemed unimaginable, with no end in sight. Each exhalation became a mighty effort to surrender my fear as I attempted once more to create a calm mind. Hearing my struggle, Michele returned to help me and suggested that I view the pain as an opening, a form of release rather than as something negative. Again the wave of pain subsided, but even this new low remained near peak level. After gaining control of my breathing I again asked for some space to work with the pain on my own.

The more I tried to still my thoughts, however, the more my efforts seemed to dredge up new causes for anxiety. Images of emergency rooms and scalpels merged with fears about lack of health insurance and expensive hospital bills. Where was my yoga practice now, when I needed it most? Why could I not control my own mind after so many years of asana and meditation? In the next instant the pain obliterated all distractions. It literally felt as if somebody had rammed the barrel of a bazooka against my right groin and pulled the trigger. Unable to even cry out, all I could do was lie in bed and squirm in agony. My breath was reduced to a shallow rasp as I reached again and again for some vestige of mental will, some shred of discipline that would allow me to regain control. At this moment Michele entered carrying a piece of paper. Seeing my inner convulsions, she remained calm and lay down on the bed beside me. "I don't know where this is from," she said. "It just came a minute ago through e-mail. I think it's for you." She handed me the paper. Something about the writing reached out to me just enough so that I could focus on the words that were now before me:

> *You are what all happenings happen in.*
> *What happens must happen, so remain unaffected as Peace.*
> *Be peaceful and this peace will spread.*
> *What rises from Peace is Peace and*
> *what rises from confusion is confusion.*
> *So be peace and give this to the Universe*
> *it is all you should do*
> *Even thinking "I am Peace" disturbs this Peace,*
> *So just be Quiet, Be as you are.*
>
> *—Papaji*

Halfway through reading the quote I began to cry. By the last word I found myself sobbing uncontrollably. For a brief moment the pain in my groin increased beyond all imagination. I could not think. What happened next happened so fast, with such force and velocity that I literally had no time to cry out. The pain in my groin became like a giant spider with steel legs puncturing my lower abdomen from the inside out. In the blink of an eye the spider withdrew its steel talons one by one and then completely dissolved. I drew in a shuddering gasp as the grip on my inguinal canal was released. The relief was instantaneous, so sharp and immediate that I could not move. The pain was completely gone. The vacuum left by the pain's sudden exit was so abrupt that for an instant it felt worse than the pain itself. I reached down to my groin and felt nothing but smooth skin and firm muscle without a lingering trace of tenderness. The rock-hard bulge of flesh had completely vanished. A sweet joy welled up from the very core of my being. Overcome with relief, my sobbing melted into deep spontaneous laughter. I floated in the experience of surrender, riding waves of grace and wonder. At that moment I could not find a care about anything that was happening to me, for I was beyond care, I was caring itself.

Michele watched this transformation with wide eyes. "It's gone, it's gone, it's gone," I told her as soon as I could speak. She hugged me and began to cry. A palpable feeling of unconditional release saturated the room. "It's gone," I cried out again, continuing to rub the flat area of my groin that only seconds before had felt like it was about to explode.

> śruta anumána prajñábhyām anyavisayā viśeśarthatvāt
> tajjah samskārah anya samskāra pratibandhī
> tasyāpi nirodhe sarva nirodhāt nirbijah samadhih

> When we see the inherent truth and beauty in whatever lies before us without the analytical knowledge that comes from books or teachings or paths, this is the beginning of Truth itself. Enjoyment of this sublime wisdom is like a beacon that obliterates the residue of all physical and mental action, bringing relief from all desires. When even the enjoyment by the mind of Truth itself is surrendered, one's consciousness becomes seedless and blissful union is experienced without separation or dependence on another.
>
> —Yoga Sutras (I. 49–51)

The word *guru* comes from Sanskrit, the ancient language of yoga. The term *gu* means "darkness." *Ru* means "light." The word *guru* means "that which takes us from darkness to light." After months of open struggle I had not found the answer to my Guru Question, yet somehow an answer had found me.

The magic of that healing moment when I received the Papaji quote from such an unexpected channel at exactly the right time was for me the arrival of the guru. In the moment of receiving that e-mail, all boundaries dissolved. It no longer mattered to me whether the guru was a revered spiritual master, a chronic illness, or the guy who cuts me off during rush hour. In that moment the experience of oneness was a reality and not some abstract mental concept or destination. And I was healed. I was whole. I was one.

The universe has at its disposal unlimited means of coordination, communication, and expression, all of it available to remind us of who we truly are. As much as I knew in my head about the ancient scriptures and multiple teachings, it was the experience of blissful union that helped me to truly understand what I now perceive as a response to my burning Guru Question. The universe provided the opportunity for vivekakhyati in a momentary burst of infinite possibility, or samadhi. In this moment of realization, I experienced the peace and freedom I so desired from my own mind. When help comes, I learned, accept it. Bless it with love and let it bless me with love and then move on when it is time, without regret or attachment.

Two men rest under a tree after a long week of digging dry wells beneath a clear summer sky. One man who keeps digging the same hole deeper and deeper proclaims that his is the best way to dig a well. The second man, who digs many shallow holes, argues with equal force that his is the best way to find water. Their discussion grows louder. The two voices carry across the dry landscape into the ears of an approaching traveler.

"Pardon me, but I could not help overhearing your conversation," the traveler says, not wanting to eavesdrop.

The two men stop arguing long enough look at the stranger, a woman dressed in the orange robes of an ascetic. "Then maybe you can help us," the first man addresses the traveler. "Who do you think is right about the best way to dig a well?"

"I am not an expert in these matters," the woman answers.

"But you must have an opinion?"

The traveler offers a slight bow. "I would not choose one or the other method."

"What are you talking about?" the second man asks.

"Either way," the traveler replies, "are you not each still standing in a hole?"

The original story, as I understand it now, has changed. There is nothing to try for and nothing to do. Nowhere to go and nothing to figure out. It is about being. The more we dig, the more we try and struggle to reach something, the further it moves away from us.

When we journey with a guru and hold that guru as separate from ourselves, we are still experiencing samskara, or duality, whether we are following one guru or many gurus. On the other extreme, it is important not to isolate by seeking "one's own" truth. This is still separation, the separation of avidya or ego, which splits our awareness away from the divine orchestration that is the true state of yoga or unity.

All great masters have had eventually to make a break from the familiar footsteps of those who came before them in order to discover their unique paths. This includes all of us, for we are all great masters. Our own doubt is the only thing that stops us from knowing that this is true. This doubt is the darkness from which we are led into the light of true knowing. Our light of experience is the only thing that we can truly share with all of creation. It is up to us to give this light to the universe.

subtle alchemy
Gladys Swan

Though I have practiced yoga in various places and circumstances over the years, much of the pleasure and benefit of doing
so has come about during my summers in Maine. Then I was free
from the responsibilities of teaching and other pressures and
was living with my family in a cabin on a lake in the woods—no
plumbing, electricity, or telephone. At the end of the semester we
piled into the car, the five of us, my husband and I, two kids, and
a golden retriever named Frito, and drove the twelve hundred
miles to where the towns grew smaller and farther apart, the

traffic diminished, and the woods took over. In north-central Maine, twenty-four miles from the nearest town, we turned off onto an unmarked dirt road, worked our heavily laden vehicle over the rocks and were *there*.

There meant putting away our watches and letting time flow as it would. The day came with bird twitter at first light, mist rising from the lake, its surface like silk, then wind ruffling it into chains of dazzle. The course of the day was measured by the way light moved through the trees and illumined certain patches of grass. The loons took over in the evenings with the rising of the moon. Unconsciously we gave ourselves to the natural rhythms of the experience of being there. As we became absorbed in our environment, first discovering, then rediscovering each year flower and berry, the signs of animal life around us, catching glimpses of deer and moose, fox, and coyote, and very rarely, bear, our previous concerns—the politics of academic life, the frustrations that came with work, personal problems—simply fell away. It took about a week to reach what we came to recognize as "the state of Maine." It seemed a different quality of consciousness, and it came with a greater intensity of being. The least activity, like watching the light on the lake, was fully significant. Food took on a special savor. The moment seemed full, and precious. Even the black flies and deer flies and mosquitoes and spiders and mice and bats that shared the space seemed to belong to the experience. In other words, I began to be aware that the life I led during the rest of the year was not the only potential. Other states of consciousness existed that one could open oneself to.

Through swimming and walking and handling a canoe, I came increasingly to the pleasures of physical activity. Yoga added another dimension. Along with maintaining a kind of suppleness, doing the asanas allowed me to begin a dialogue with my body, to put myself into various positions and take in the subtle psychology of being in them. Suddenly you discover that you can do something you hadn't managed before; you can hold a pose for a longer period. You appreciate the sensations of tension and release. To enter both physically and imaginatively into those states of tension, relaxation, balance, motion, and stability the asanas call for provides a certain focus and awareness that might otherwise remain unconscious. The limits you always assumed would never change begin to dissolve. Paying attention to breathing, going into a deeper state of concentration, allowed me to step outside the usual time-bound activities, the fractured surfaces of daily life, the continual pressures of measuring up, being useful, responding to the demands of work or family. Though I wasn't aware of it at the time, I was helping create a space where I could simply be. This seemed to offer a route toward what Yeats calls "the unity of being," and Blake's sense that one doesn't *have* a body; one *is* a body.

Despite the emphasis on sex in this culture and its exploitation in the media, I find a number of tendencies that militate against the simple acceptance of one's physical being: the notions of failure attached to infirmity or the lack of physical beauty or the inability to make the team. Not that physical beauty shouldn't be appreciated or that physical prowess and athletic skill shouldn't be admired. But it is difficult to locate avenues that foster self-acceptance, beginning with one's physical nature, a simple acceptance of what allows us to exist in the world. I have come across a number of people whose response to nudity is a sense of shame and the feeling that the naked body should be covered up as fast as possible. As I prepare an exhibit for my artwork in a local historical society gallery, I am told not to hang any nudes–this would require too much explanation to school-children. Such attitudes, to my mind, foster the division between body and spirit. I believe that yoga can offer a basis for self-esteem, a way of putting one in touch with the central fact of all existence, the act of breathing, and give value to the body as the incarnation of being. This can lead to an inwardness that is not a neurotic self-absorption; quite the contrary.

The word *yoga* means "unity," and it appears that when we are freed of the various distractions and illusions that beguile us, we are open to the unity that we are and that makes us part of everything that exists. "Everything that lives is holy," Blake wrote. Among the asanas are those that suggest other forms of life: the tree, the bird, the frog, the cobra, the scorpion, the cow, the lion, the camel, as though by putting ourselves in certain postures, we can enter imaginatively into the energies that create these forms and capture something of both essence and symbol. Taking the pose of the cat, for instance, putting myself down on the floor as a four-footed creature, gives me a moment as I arch and lower my back to try to enter into what has always fascinated me about that interesting animal: the combination of playfulness and wildness, independence and affection, a talent for ultimate repose as well as the ability to concentrate with extended patience, poised like a spring in readiness–all held together with a wonderful grace of movement and a real pleasure in being what it is. Perhaps by such an act of imagination, one comes to a certain empathy, a recognition that the breath we breathe in and out is shared by all forms of life.

It has been beneficial to me to allow myself to try to engage the various forms–insect and bird, plant and animal. The glimpses of bird and animal life have felt like a kind of blessing from some part of nature revealing itself. One is given a continuing invitation to look around and see what's there, even to develop seeing into a kind of art. One summer I spent my time searching out and identifying all the wildflowers in the vicinity–some seventy-five in all. It was not just a question of finding them, but of looking at them closely in terms of the color, the arrangement of the petals, the shape of the leaves, the relation of leaf to flower. It took concentration. Now I look forward each summer to certain presences: the two towering white pines behind the privy; the swallows that nest in the eaves of the cabin; the frogs down in the swamp, where the bull-head lilies and pickerelweed bloom, where the fallen dead trees become nurse logs for all kinds of plants in a continuation of life that suggests that nothing is final. Over the years my sense of the way individual elements form a recurring cycle has deepened.

All of this is not to say that a certain set of circumstances or experiences is required to gain the sense of a center. I'm simply recording what occurred in my case. You don't have to flee to the Maine woods or run away anywhere to locate the inner being, since it's always there. It can open up to recognition in one's own backyard or on a city street. I can say now that "the readiness is all." The Maine woods is perhaps a good metaphor, like Thoreau's *Walden,* something that points in the direction of living more deliberately, of determining what is necessary for one's life, what fosters its best potentials. Concentrating on one's breath in a quiet room is finally all that's necessary to confirm an underlying reality.

It may be that the practice of yoga has helped create in me a basic attitude, a kind of openness and receptivity both to inward and outer experience, and beyond that, a capacity for letting go. At times I have had to pause in the middle of the exercises to go and write down the images that came to me or important ideas connected to what I was writing. When I am in the midst of creating something, a certain magnetism seems to draw ideas and images to the work at hand. I recognize the necessity for being open to them. And so with outward experience. I find it easier to let go of ideas, even cherished ideas, that no longer serve. Several years ago when I developed a stress-related illness, I practiced yoga daily, using the tapes of Jon Kabat-Zinn. They were particularly helpful in creating a state of relaxation, releasing pressure, and letting go of negative thinking.

I'm convinced that the capacity to concentrate and to let go of the ego gives a special dimension to one's work, whatever that work is, whether it's laying carpet or walking the high wire. I'm speaking of the ability to forget everything except the work itself. My dentist, passionately dedicated to the practice of dentistry, once said to me as he was putting in a crown, "Sometimes I get so involved when I'm working, I almost forget to breathe." Recently when I was volunteering with Circus Flora in St. Louis, I asked one of the members of the Flying Wallendas what he thought about when he was walking the high wire. He told me there was no room for thought–it was a matter of putting one foot in front of the other. The extraordinary risk requires complete concentration. "Not a place for daydreaming," he said.

My own work has been as a writer and visual artist. Whether or not yoga has directly influenced the practice of the particular arts I have engaged in, it has certainly offered a certain touchstone by which I can compare the two realms and determine certain relationships. My first clue came some years ago when I was working in ceramics at Purdue University. I had never undertaken anything before that depended so much on manual skill and coordination; it took me far longer than most to learn to throw a pot. Working alongside me those nights that sometimes extended to two or three in the morning was a potter who threw wonderful forms with great ease while I labored over mine, with many failures. His name was Ron, and he'd lost a couple of fingers on his right hand and the joint of his left thumb in some horrible industrial accident when he was a factory worker. He'd had to relearn how to throw and somehow managed to use his mutilated thumb to advantage and to compensate for the missing fingers. Often I'd say to him, "Ron, that's a fine pot," to which he'd respond with a little grunt of acknowledgment and carry on. He made no such comments about my productions—until one evening I threw a pot that evoked his admiration. I set it aside, and to my astonishment everyone who came into the room stopped to admire it. "Who made that pot?" they wanted to know. What were they responding to? I wanted to ask. What was the difference between this and other pots I had thrown? I was mystified.

It was years later that I came to some idea. What I believe had happened was this: Somehow I had relaxed my efforts to "get it right," and through the space outside my control something had flowed through my hands into the clay, something beyond what I knew, something unconscious and deeply intuitive, which apparently touched a chord in other people. Or perhaps I had done what my drawing teacher, Curt Stocking, used to refer to as "working on the point of time." What I think he meant was entering a state in which nothing intervenes between one's conscious presence and the object of contemplation, a moment stripped of ego. In that state the accepted definitions of reality, the social, moral, and aesthetic judgments that usually operate fall away, clearing the path for other insights and sources of inspiration. Perhaps this statement by the painter Edouard Vuillard also sheds light on the phenomenon: "If in raising my eyes to a painting or to nature I *will* to observe, I fall into falsity. One observes, one cannot will [oneself] to observe. The emotion contained therein (observation) alone can give—is the primary condition of—a work of art, before the spirit of method and the practical intelligence that are born of the selfsame spirit that undergoes this emotion."

Keats's term *negative capability* applies here as well, his statement that the poetical character "has no self—it is every thing and nothing—It has no character—it enjoys light and shade; it lives in gusto, be it foul or fair, high or low, rich or poor, mean or elevated—It has as much delight in conceiving an Iago as an Imogene." And, finally, in the terms of dance, a similar state is necessary to reach the ecstatic, a state that dance historian Curt Sachs, quoting the German writer Beck, speaks of as the "unburdening of the will." According to Beck, "The movements are executed automatically without the intervention of the self. Thus the consciousness of self disappears completely and is lost in the primitive consciousness."

As I have worked over the years, I have come to know more and more the thrill of being in that state. Two or three hours pass in a single moment. And from that moment comes the sense of discovery and wonder I feel when I look at the image I have painted or what I've written. It seems as though someone else must have done it. I have no knowledge of how I came to it. This is not to denigrate technique and craft and the exercise of one's critical sense. They are necessary to help create the vessel, to open the way to make the other possible, but they cannot displace it. As Curt Stocking used to say, "Realization is as important as practice." You could practice twice as much, he told me once, but you wouldn't necessarily improve at twice the rate, though some improvement might take place. I have come to recognize the truth of his statement. I know of certain points, fortuitous moments, when I knew my work had moved to a different plane. But not because of anything I planned.

I have found, in concentrating on the work, in entering a state where the work exists as an object of contemplation, a sense of authenticity and freedom. It has allowed me to accept the intrinsic demands of a form for its fulfillment, to let the form emerge from the materials. This has allowed a kind of spontaneity and at the same time prevented me from easy solutions. It has created some difficulties as well—particularly in finding an audience and avenues of publication. But perhaps, as one looks at the creative source, that is not the point.

For me, the sense of timelessness in time, the moment stripped of ego, is what relates the practice of yoga to other practices—T. S. Eliot's moment in the rose garden, a moment when it is possible to apprehend a reality underlying what exists in time, the sense of "the still point of the turning world," which he sees as the fundamental religious experience that cuts across all religions. It seems to me that the difference between the practice of yoga and the practice of an art is that the first allows one to clear away the clutter that stands in the way of reaching that moment, to still the chattering of the mind, while the second is concerned with creating those images that point toward various states of insight, emotion, and apprehension. The loss of self in the absolute, the ultimate state of concentration, is the path of yoga. The aim of the arts is expression. As artist Dorothy McCray, another of my teachers, has put it: "Art is the expression of the astonishment at the moment-by-moment experience of being." The effort can be enhanced—perhaps ultimately it is made possible—by touching a similar point at some deep level, to get beyond the surfaces of society and convention, the demands of daily life, to touch their hidden springs and remind us of the sources that feed us.

corpse pose
A. B. Emrys

Savasana, the most difficult yoga pose: Lie on the floor on your back, arms open, palms up, legs slightly apart. Keep lying there. Watch yourself breathe. Watch your thoughts fold and unfold. Watch your breath some more.

That's it.

I've only fallen asleep once in three years. Often I yawn, reaching up my jaw, biting air. Often my lower back throws out on the last forward bend. Sometimes my teacher brings a bolster to put under my knees, and then I float backwards. Every kind of thing goes around my head.

*

My dad doesn't ever lie down flat anymore. I see at the hospital that his bed is cranked up, and at home a complicated mound of pillows props him. Mama sees me notice this, and hastens to explain that he breathes better this way. He concentrates on his breathing as hard as I do on words. Right now every breath takes as much effort as he's got. He struggles one by one, not to suck it in but to expand his lungs and accept it. He gasps exactly like the fish he used to catch, gills working on nothing, bodies flopping, trying to swim away. He drinks the oxygen feed but little of it hits the bloodstream. He's sweating and exhausted from breathing. I've never seen him this bad, though mama says she has, plenty of times. "You're just having a bad day," she says to him. "I'm having kind of a bad day, too."

I breathe shallowly around my parents, as though breathing will call attention to myself. Outside the hospital, looking for my car in the parking lot, I gulp huge breaths of dry air. Back at the house I do my daily yoga on the carport driveway. Hot cement grinds the bottom of my feet. I try to stay with my breath, let it tell me when to loosen a pose, when to go deeper, when to move out of it. I sit outside a while too. Mrs. M., an acquaintance, stops by to ask how my dad's doing. She looks at me oddly. What were those weird moves I was doing, maybe, or Why are my parents here old and alone? I sit some more, until I see I'm avoiding going inside.

Inside the house I lived in from eighth grade through junior year at State I know I will find:
—Bags of coupons clipped from newspapers and magazines. Clipped neatly as a child learns to cut, not torn out jagged like I do. Literally bags of them, armfuls. All expired. She won't let me throw any away. "Those have information I need." She sees to cut with the sides of her macula, turning her head like a bird. While she was with my dad at the hospital, I said to my sister, "I'm going to get rid of some of these old ones. She'll never know the difference." At that instant the phone rang. She'd found the pay phones

and punched by touch. "Don't move any of my coupons," she said. "I need those."

–Faded, random pseudopaintings collected god knows why, all dusty, some strung with cobwebs. The huge photo of my sister fat and string-haired in velvet, me with tortured hair and an ugly slate-blue dress I can still feel clutch my throat, has roach eggs crusted down one side of it like barnacles. I can't vacuum them off, and can't stand to touch them. My sister Les says, "We're going to burn that after they're gone, aren't we?"

–Under the stove top, a quarter-inch of grease from bacon and fried eggs they must eat every morning, or die. I scrape it off with a spoon.

–On the head of my dad's bed, my old bookcase headboard I never kept books in, his rifle, loaded. A last stand at the homestead against all comers. As I clean under his bed, the vacuum sucks up a shell. He had a pistol, too, which they believe one of the ambulance attendants stole when they came into the bedroom to lift him onto a gurney. Either that or it's lost under the strata of clothes, unmatched bedding, Christmas ornaments, and sheer stuff that surrounds his bed. I clean the dust from his guitar and lean it next to the gun.

–Dozens of pots and pans under the counters. Depression consumer thinking: Don't throw anything away, ever; buy new ones, too. About half the pans have food dried in them. I clean some and throw some out.

–The wash bucket in the yard. Something's wrong with the machine. They claim it requires a sewer hookup. I offer to pay for it. My brother-in-law, the licensed plumber, offers to install the new machine. My mother washes their clothes with a stick, the way her mother did before they moved to town. She hangs the soapy clothes and rinses them with the hose. This proves something to her. It proves something to us too.

The house itself Les, her husband, and I discuss when we're alone. Bring in a work crew, strip out the old carpet and the furniture, fumigate, polish the tile, repaint. Our mother tells me later she'll live on there, sorting everything "if he dies—but I've seen him this bad plenty of times." The house, she says, will be sold to send my nephews to college. "I've promised it to those little children," she says, a tremor vibrating on "promise," Another night, angry, she says she'll move "back to the country. I understand country people. They don't do you like these people in town."

The hospital ward my dad's in consists entirely of old people propped up in beds trying not to die yet, maybe secretly hoping to. I go up in the wheelchair-sized elevator, and exit right into corpse rehearsal row. They're all gray faced and white haired, paper skinned, shrunken, helpless. Tubes attach to their heads, hands, forearms, under sheets out of sight. I see all this in flinching glances walking past quickly, turn into my dad's room past the old man who's now watching TV instead of his breath, and see my dad's face, the oxygen line like a water buffalo's nose lead. Eating breakfast has left him panting again.

My mother slept on a sort of cot pushed in by the sink. The hospital would bring a courtesy meal for her on request, but instead she picks at the remains of my dad's meal while he breathes. She's wearing an electric purple sweater and a stained pair of slacks. Even to me, remembering decades of messy housekeeping and money confusions, the weekly screaming panics, the ritualized craziness that passed for reality, they look neglected. Tonight on the phone my daughter will promise to shoot me before I get to this point. She means the hospital row. We both know I won't end in a cobweb of paranoia. You think I'm exaggerating here, I bet.

When Les shows up to sit a while, I drive Mama back to the house. This time I get her to wait in front of the hospital for me to bring the car up. There's a trolley that takes people around to cars, but she won't ride it. After I pick her up and she's got me safely lined up on the road, her voice shifts into the holy tone she uses to speak of illness. "Your sister is developing heart trouble," she says.

Daddy's dying, and she comes out with this. I ask the key question: "Has she seen a doctor?"

My mother leans closer. "I could tell when I touched her hand," she says.

When I try to explain my family to newer friends, they think it's old age, but age has only made it more pitiable. I didn't see my parents for ten years at one point, barely spoke to them after Mama began calling up and diagnosing from my daughter's voice that she had diphtheria, the same way she once decided I had asthma, allergies, needed my tonsils out, even though the second opinions always disagreed in front of me. She does it now with my dad. At home, after I've seen him sweating to breathe, calling out to God to take him, she'll eventually tell me that he doesn't really feel much pain–"It's just the stress. What he really needs is a very mild tranquilizer." Les has no sympathy for him. "Now he knows," she says, "what it was like for us growing up."

This hypertext blows through my head in a nanosecond, and I fall back on the doctor. No matter what else she says, I just suggest Les should see a doctor. Eventually Mama goes off into complaints about my dad's doctors, and I concentrate on driving. She has taken pains to compliment me on my driving–"I think you've turned out to be a very capable driver"–while managing to imply that there was some doubt.

When I'm moving through the poses, warrior one, two, three, or Surya Namaskara, lunging and bowing, my mind calms. I think in my body, move by move. It's difficult enough that I don't have spare conscious attention for any little worries, any little bits of the past to chew on. I just move, up, down, forward extension, upward hands, standing cobra. I've just enough breath to do it. My leg muscles tremble after a few minutes, so that tree pose, leg on opposite thigh, sways and falls over. But my mind is calm.

This is how my mother lives moment to moment. Cook the bacon, put the dishes on to soak, sit down and nap a few minutes, sort of wash dishes, get out frozen dinners for lunch, same as after breakfast, wash some clothes in the bucket. When she's moving or asleep, she's okay. Meanwhile my dad lies there coaxing air. Corpse pose is the most difficult because you're not in motion. There's no external movement to block the stream. The conscious mind is a spectacle, and it morphs like dreams.

Friday night I walk out into the hall with the doctor after he comes by on rounds. He's young, focused, articulate. He thinks my dad has only a few days. Mama won't discuss funeral arrangements with me for more than two minutes. She has no idea what he wants, and won't bring it up to him, as though it's unlucky. Saturday morning I look up parlors in the phone book. The one they favor, for reasons unknown, is in the old part of town, and to get there, I have to cross the rodeo parade. Les and her husband and kids went to watch it. I remember seeing it when I was in grade school, palominos with silver saddle trimmings flashing in the sun, bright bay horses and red banners, ritzy cowboy pomp. Now I just drive till I find a cross street.

There's no fanfare at the parlor. It's quiet as a—well, you know. They also speak in awed voices, as though their very jobs are near-death experiences. I acquire a maroon folder with prices. Ma and Pa have been fairly accurate in their guesstimate. The money for his funeral is at the moment in a desk drawer in a cashier's check that they've had for months. I really don't know if he'd prefer to be buried in the West he loves, or in the Ozarks of his boyhood. Staring at the cheaply printed pages, I start thinking of what might go on his tombstone. I think it should be a line from "El Paso," his favorite Marty Robbins song. He played the tape of it in the car the last time I was here that he could drive. Maybe "I can see Rosie's Cantina below." Singing in my head, I stuff the sheets in the spiffy textured folder and drive back through the now empty streets. Mama makes me bury it in the hall table drawer.

For yoga, I am to watch my mind, but any time I'm around Mama, I end up watching hers. I've never seen the lake of her mind quiet. Always there's a storm coming on, raging, or blowing away. The storms always come from the same direction, the past. So much she hated, wished she'd done differently, can't forget. She half-believes she was adopted, a way of explaining the way her parents indulged her much younger sister. She can't stand any of her family for long, insists always that blood relatives are all you've got, and has made it true. She dislikes little kids, and wished aloud in front of my sister and I that she'd had a son. When I draw her attention toward one bout of worry weather, she leaps to another. I feel again, as I did for nearly two decades, as though I'm in her mind, the world is her mind, and all I can do is watch it leapfrog reality.

Today Mama brought the bills for my dad to write checks, as he always has done, even in the years she, too, taught full-time. Halfway through he has to lie back (still mostly upright) and rest. Like a complete idiot or a normal person, I suggest that they institute direct deposit and automatic deduction, which I have for my paycheck and the mortgage. "You'd better check every month and make sure they put the right amount in," she says. Even Daddy draws enough breath to concur: "And another thing"–breathing–"they take it out right away"–breathing–"better make sure you have enough to cover it." No help, they mean. We have to suffer. They understand perfectly that existence is anguish, but being Americans, they want credit for it. They want an audience for it. I realize that acutely after my sister and her family leave and I'm the only one still in the ringside seat.

Every night my mother says, "Why don't you just take a break and do something for fun?" as though I've come here for a vacation. The fourth night I go for Mexican food at a diner, and then to a theater where I watch Jamie Lee frag half-mechanical aliens who consider humans a virus. When I'm back at the house reading *Slaves in the Family* and making puns on the title, Mama calls with a list of trivial errands for me to start in the morning. Among other things, she needs a bigger washtub.

My dad comes home on Monday because the hospital expects him to die. There isn't anything else they can do, and he's taking up a bed. At home with a leaky catheter bag, he so miserable I expect him to pick up the gun. He yells and curses, and finally passes out a while. I sleep with earplugs that night, and I'm the only one who sleeps much. My mother has laid at the foot of his bed on a quilt much of the night, waking him frequently to make sure he's still alive. By that night he's talked his doctor into twenty-four hours in the emergency ward. He's there when I leave the next day, getting whatever he wants. I say good-bye as if for good. My sister told him to say hi to granddad for her, as she can't remember him. The last time he had been hospitalized, his father appeared, beckoning.

In fact, I talked to him a few days ago, more than a year later. This is messy nonfiction, not the satisfying plots I've spent much of my free lifetime reading. As I drove to Phoenix and stayed in an old motel with only one lamp in its large room and a phone that kept falling out of the wall, my dad came home again and this time stabilized. While I was rushing back from Omaha to my job, he caught his breath. Maybe the drugs finally kicked in enough, maybe his bowels cleared enough. My theory is that he recovered because he got so mad at the hospice people: Nobody's taking over his decisions, deathbed or no. He was briefly hospitalized again five months later, this time airlifted to Phoenix where doctors installed a pacemaker.

The week I spent with them was anticlimax for us all. My dad, who'd been groaning aloud, "Just take me now," settled down to enjoying basketball games and the occasional Western. He's rehearsed for the end, but being unable to get a breath is torture every time, and that likely is how he'll die. My mom lost her audience and went back to moving unminded through her tasks, punctuated with phone calls. Les and I went back to our lives with little to give others for some time. It was rehearsal for all of us. This wasn't the big one; that will improv out of the blue, maybe when we least expect it.

For the past year, whenever I try to think about when and how next, my mind blanks. I watch it do this over and over. My repeated offers to hook up the sewer, stage-manage legal details, major cleaning, or any other relevant item, my parents have entirely refused. My mother says I should just come home for a visit. My dad doesn't say much at a time, especially if the humidity's high.

Visiting my parents, it's always corpse pose practice. Watch them suffer. Watch the anxiety shift to a new topic. Watch it some more. Corpse pose is my relationship to them. I know their ultimate causes and excuses. The depression. The Second World War. Changing up to middle class without a guidebook. A bad marriage till death divorces. Moving away from your family and having your kids do the same. Decades of gender muddle, career muddle, retirement muddle. It's their generation, which seemed to have stopped taking in new information around 1950. It's their karma. All their pathos is tinged with choice. They have arrived down a glaringly yellow-brick road their feet skipped onto long ago.

My mother called today, to say the past is repeating. My dad's been in the hospital three weeks, in a "transitional care" ward. We all know where the transition's heading. She wants me to come scrub the house, witness the misery, but they still won't discuss death arrangements. It's my karma too, so I must have choices. Beyond Savasana is upright meditation. We practiced it in class with mental exercises. One was to walk from home to class in the mind. I found I couldn't turn corners in my mind. When I got to the corner I just kept going, or actually swung my body left trying to turn. Finally I grabbed the whole street around the corner and swung it in front of me, or me in front of it. Then I went on to the next corner. I'll call my sister tonight, and see which of us is going when. Meantime, I do lots of warrior poses, my favorites, so balanced and strong that I can hold the illusion minutes at a time.

contributors

Janet Bowdan and Roz Peters are cousins who have been writing to each other between America and England for twenty-five years. Janet Bowdan is an associate professor of English at Western New England College in Springfield, Massachusetts, where she teaches composition, creative writing, British literature, and a comparative cultures course on Australia and New Zealand. She has published poems in *American Poetry Review, Denver Quarterly, Hawaii Review, Crazyhorse, Verse, Colorado Review,* and other journals. Her poem "The Year" appears in *Best American Poetry 2000.* Roz Peters has been studying yoga for twelve

years, Ashtanga yoga for nine. She has studied with K. Pattabhi
Jois and has taught yoga since 1994.

Samantha Dunn was raised in northern New Mexico and spent
years in Australia and France. She is a widely published American journalist contributing to a number of magazines and newspapers in the United States, including the *Los Angeles Times, L.A.*

*Weekly, Details, Cosmopolitan, Premiere, Men's Fitness, Yoga Jour-
nal, Shape, Shape Cooks, Live!, Speak, InStyle, Bikini,* and *Condé
Nast Women's Sports+ Fitness.* Her first novel, *Failing Paris* (1999),
is short-listed for the PEN Center West PEN/Faulkner Award.

A. B. Emrys's writing has appeared in many journals, including *Portland, Prairie Schooner,* and *Paragraph,* and in the
anthologies *Sacred Ground: Writings about Home* and *Air Fish.*
She continues to practice yoga and writing, often as metaphors
for each other.

Vyaas Houston is the founder and director of the American Sanskrit Institute. He studied Sanskrit with Ramamurti Mishra and
at Columbia University, where he received his M.A. After teaching Sanskrit and yoga for more than fifteen years, he discovered
in 1987 a successful method for teaching Sanskrit based on the
yoga model of Patanjali's Yoga Sutras. His Sanskrit training has
provided thousands of people with the opportunity to discover
their own unique relationship with Sanskrit. He is also the
author of *Sanskrit by Cassette,* and has recorded and translated
many Sanskrit classics.

Elizabeth Kadetsky began studying Iyengar yoga in 1984. A graduate of the M.F.A. fiction program at the University of California
at Irvine, she has published fiction and journalism in *Santa
Monica Review, Greensboro Review, Village Voice, Ms.,* and many
other publications. "Coming Apart in Pune" is part of a memoir
in progress based on her experiences studying yoga as a Ful-
bright scholar in India.

Judith Hanson Lasater, Ph.D., physical therapist, is an internationally known yoga teacher and the author of *Relax and Renew: Restful Yoga for Stressful Times* and *Living Your Yoga: Finding the Spiritual in Everyday Life.* She was a founder of *Yoga Journal* and writes frequently for *Natural Health* and national magazines about health and yoga. She is the mother of three fascinating young adults. Ms. Lasater can be reached at www.judithlasater.com.

Jeff Martens, a writer and yoga teacher, is cofounder of the YogaVision International Yoga Conference and directs the YogaVision yoga program at Arizona State University.

Lois Nesbitt began practicing yoga as a teenager. She resumed her studies as an adult, and has been practicing Ashtanga yoga regularly for seven years, under Eddie Stern of the Patanjali Yoga Shala in New York City and Sri K. Pattabhi Jois of Mysore, India. She has been certified by and has taught at Yoga Zone and Integral Yoga Institute in New York City and is currently undergoing certification in Anusara yoga under John Friend. She lives in New York and summers in the Hamptons.

Robert Perkins is a noted documentary filmmaker and writer. His books include *Talking to Angels, Into the Great Solitude,* and *Against Straight Lines.* His next film, *The Crocodile River,* will take him down the great, green, greasy Limpopo River in southern Africa. He received the Ingram Merrill Award for Creativity.

Adrian M. S. Piper is a svanistha brahmacharin, conceptual artist, and professor of philosophy at Wellesley College. She is the recipient of numerous awards and fellowships in art and philosophy, and her artwork is in many important collections. Two retrospectives are traveling nationally and internationally. She is the author of articles on metaethics and Kant, as well as *Out of Order, Out of Sight: Selected Writings in Meta-Art and Art Criti-*

cism 1967–1992. Her project in Kantian metaethics, *Rationality and the Structure of the Self,* is nearing completion.

Stanley Plumly is the author of six poetry collections and recipient of numerous awards, including a Guggenheim Fellowship and three National Endowment for the Arts Awards. His most recent book is *Now That My Father Lies Down Beside Me: New and Selected Poems, 1970–2000.* He is Distinguished University Professor at the University of Maryland. He studies yoga with Judith Lyon in Bethesda, Maryland.

Gladys Swan's works include *On the Edge of the Desert* (short fiction), 1979; *Carnival for the Gods* (novel), 1986; *Of Memory and Desire* (short fiction), 1989; *Do You Believe in Cabeza de Vaca?* (short fiction), 1991; and *Ghost Dance: A Play of Voices* (novel), 1992.

Reetika Vazirani is the author of *White Elephants* (1996), which won a Barnard New Women Poets Prize, and *World Hotel* (2002). Educated at Wellesley College and the University of Virginia, she is a contributing and advisory editor of *Callaloo.* Her new poems appear in *Best American Poetry 2000, Paris Review,* and others.

Alison West was born in Paris and educated in France and England. She returned to New York for her undergraduate work in Russian and graduate work in art history, while continuing to study dance. She began yoga in Munich while writing her dissertation. After a brief teaching stint at Barnard and a National Endowment for the Humanities grant, she turned to choreography, and finally to yoga full-time. She teaches independently in Soho. In 1998, Cambridge University Press published her book *From Pigalle to Preault: Neoclassicism and the Sublime in French Sculpture, 1760–1840.*

acknowledgments

My thanks first and foremost to Amy Caldwell at Beacon Press for her support and love of this book. Thank you also to Dave Oliver, my yoga teacher of ten years, and to Melissa Pritchard, my writing teacher. You have both taught me so much. Thanks to my parents and daughters–unknowing fodder for my introduction–to Genevieve Hangen, Teresa Koneche, Natalie Jeremijenko, Margaret Bates, Barbara Grubel, Seane Corn, Charlie Scott, the community at Yoga Source, and the faculty and staff of Virginia Commonwealth University Department of Dance and Choreography. Most especially my thanks to all the writers, yoga practitioners, and teachers who supported this book and contributed to it. Thank you also to Chris English, with whom I began and continue down the yoga path.